So then because thou art lukewarm,

and neither cold nor hot,

I will spew thee out of my mouth.

Revelation 3:16

YOU NEED TO KNOW...
THE HEALTH MESSAGE

Do you not know that you are God's temple and that God's Spirit dwells in you? If anyone destroys God's temple, God will destroy him, For God's temple is holy and that temple you are.
1 Corinthians 3:16-17

So, whether you eat or drink, or whatever you do, do all to the glory of God. 1 Corinthians 10:31

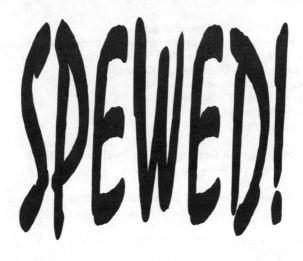

SPEWED!

How To Cast Out Lukewarm Christianity through

FASTING

and a

FASTED LIFESTYLE

Plus: Using WISDOM in Fasting

Beth M. Ley, Ph.D.

BL Publications
Detroit Lakes, MN

Library of Congress Cataloging-in-Publication Data

Ley, Beth M., 1964-
    Spued! : how to cast out lukewarm Christianity through fasting and a fasted lifestyle / Beth M. Ley.
        p. cm.
Includes bibliographical references.
    ISBN 1-890766-22-4
    1. Fasting--Religious aspects--Christianity. I. Title.

    BV5055.L48 2003
    248.4'7--dc21

                                    2003007767

Printed in the United States of America

All scriptures are taken from The King James Version of the Holy Bible unless otherwise stated.

All scripture quotations marked AMP are taken from THE AMPLIFIED BIBLE, Old Testament Copyright © 1965, 1987 by the Zondervan Corporation, Amplified New Testament Copyright © 1958, 1987 by the Lockman Foundation. used by permission.

This book is not intended as medical advice. Its purpose is solely educational. Please consult your healthcare professional for all health problems.

Credits

Cover Design: BL Publications

Proofreaders: Wendy Gordon, Betty Keller, LaDonna Schumacher, Naomi Bogda

Spiritual coverage: Wendy Gordon, Margie Frankburg, Irene Cornelius, Melvin and Carol Schultz, Pete and Bonnie Lage, Deb and Jeff Krueger, Kenneth and Stephanie Scott.

Distributed by NHL Ministries, Detroit Lakes, MN
Greater Health... God's Way

TABLE OF CONTENTS

INTRODUCTION

When God Calls a Fast

God will do whatever it takes to draw us to him. He wants a personal relationship with us. The purpose He created us was for us to have a personal relationship with Him. He wants us to spend time with Him, talk to Him, listen to Him and depend on Him for everything. He wants our obedience. Most of all, He wants to be the focus of our lives. This was number one on His list of top ten commandments given to Moses in Exodus 20:3 *Thou shalt have no other gods before me.* The bottom line is God is a jealous God. He must be first in our life.

If God is not first, He may allow circumstances to happen that will make us so miserable that we can do nothing but cry out to Him. No matter what we are going through, God is always there waiting to rescue us.

In the midst of "the trial," this may seem cruel, but in most cases if we look back on our lives and recognize the times when this may have happened, we will see what God was trying to do or teach us and it will make more sense.

Several years ago, at a time of great distress, I cried out to God, "What can I do?" He answered, "You could fast." I was quite perplexed at this answer as I was unfamiliar and unexperienced with fasting at the time.... an area neglected in my teachings and readings.

Thus began my journey of fasting, research and the inspiration of this book and all that God had to reveal to me. As much of the book is about keeping our focus on Him and off of the distractions of the world and the flesh, preparing for and writing of this book was very difficult and challenging. The learning process of grasping what God is trying to teach us can be very painful indeed.

It's in the Valleys We Grow

(Unknown Author)

Sometimes life seems hard to bear,
Full of sorrow, trouble and woe
It's then we have to remember
That it's in the valleys we grow.

If we always stayed on the mountain top
And never experienced pain,
We would never appreciate God's love
And would be living in vain.

We have so much to learn
And our growth is very slow,
Sometimes we need the mountain tops,
But it's in the valleys we grow.

We do not always understand
Why things happen as they do,
But I am very sure of one thing.
My Lord will see me through.
The little valleys are nothing
When we picture Christ on the cross
He went through the valley of death;
His victory was Satan's loss.

Forgive me Lord, for complaining
When I'm feeling so very low.
Just give me a gentle reminder
That it's in the valleys I grow.

Continue to strengthen me, Lord
And use my life each day
To share your love with others
And help them find their way.

Thank you for the valleys, Lord
For this one thing I know
The mountain tops are glorious
But it's in the valleys I grow!

After a brief introduction to fasting, I discuss why God is calling us to fast and how it affects our relationship with Him. After this I will explain the concept of lukewarmness and why God hates this so much, and fasting as it relates to our focus on God, holiness, sanctification and the power we receive from fasting.

I then discuss the significance of food and our responsibility to our bodies, as temples of the holy spirit. This is followed with practical information to help you in your journey with God in fasting. This includes very important information on how to safe guard our health. We must be wise in fasting so not to tear down our bodies. I believe this part of the book alone makes the book a worthwhile investment.

Fasting 101

A fast generally refers to the voluntary abstinence from eating food or from certain kinds of food. Fasting is an act of worship and of service unto God. Fasting can also be an act of mourning or an act of humbling and cleansing.

Fasting was a common practice among Jews and was continued among Christians. In Acts 27:9, "the fast" refers to the Day of Atonement, *Now when much time was spent, and when sailing was now dangerous, because the fast was now already past.*

This was the famous yearly fast of the Jews on the tenth day of the seventh month. It was a day to afflict the soul with fasting (about the 20th of September). This yearly fast was faithfully observed; but strangely, the only time it is mentioned in the New Testament is here in Acts, where it serves only to describe the season of the year.

And this shall be a statute for ever unto you: that in the seventh month, on the tenth day of the month, ye shall afflict your souls, and do no work at all, Whether it be one of your own country, or a stranger that sojourneth among you: For on that day shall the priest make an atonement for you, to cleanse you, that ye may be clean from all your sins before the LORD. **Leviticus 16:29-30**

There are, of course, right and wrong ways to fast, which will be covered in more detail later. The Pharisees are commonly identified as those who fasted in vain. Anna is an example of one who honored God when she fasted, and therefore, who God honored.

5

And there was one Anna, a prophetess, the daughter of Phanuel, of the tribe of Aser: she was of a great age, and had lived with a husband seven years from her virginity. And she was a widow of about fourscore and four years, which departed not from the temple, but served God with fastings and prayers night and day. **Luke 2:36-37**

Anna served God with fastings and prayers night and day, having no secular business to employ herself in. She gave up herself wholly to prayer, and not only fasted twice a week, but lived a fasted lifestyle unlike the religious exercises which others spent in eating and drinking and sleeping. She not only observed the regular hours of prayer, but prayed always night and day.

Anna was only in her twenties when her husband died and when she gave herself to this fasted lifestyle of solemn prayer serving God. We don't need to be "old" or wait until we are old, or alone and widowed to have this type of call or anointing on our life. We simply need to the the fire of God burning within us for more of God!

Anna not only did that which was good, but did it with a pure heart. Her service to God was aimed at His honor. The Pharisees fasted often, and made long prayers, but they served themselves (instead of God), and their own pride and covetousness in their fastings and prayers. (Luke 18:9-14)

God may call us to seasons of serving in various ways, and then lead us to do something else. It is important to be in constant communication with God to know what it is that He would have us doing at that particular time. We should be in constant prayer. We should never let our lives get so busy that we cannot hear God. We need to be in tune to the Spirit.

Why We Should Fast

Fasting is not required. Nowhere in the Bible does it say that we must fast. Fasting is not required for salvation. However, there are numerous times that God recommends fasting. In Joel, God tells the people to humble themselves, repent, mourn and fast. *Sanctify ye a fast, call a solemn assembly, gather the elders and all the inhabitants of the land into the house of the LORD your God, and cry unto the LORD.* **Joel 1:14**

Joel 2 highlights perhaps the most important aspects of fasting: to humble oneself, to repent and to mourn. When we repent of our sins, through the death of Jesus we are forgiven and intimacy with Him and the Father can be restored.

Therefore also now, saith the LORD, turn ye even to me with all your heart, and with fasting, and with weeping, and with mourning: And rend your heart, and not your garments, and turn unto the LORD your God: for he is gracious and merciful, slow to anger, and of great kindness, and repenteth him of the evil. Who knoweth if he will return and repent, and leave a blessing behind him; even a meat offering and a drink offering unto the LORD your God? Blow the trumpet in Zion, sanctify a fast, call a solemn assembly. **Joel 2:12-15**

If this is done, God promises to restore us: *And I will restore to you the years that the locust hath eaten, the cankerworm, and the caterpillar, and the palmerworm, my great army which I sent among you.* **Joel 2:25**

In order for God to pour out His Spirit and to bless us, we first MUST humble ourselves and repent.

God Hates Pride!

The Greek meaning of pride, Strongs #212 ala-zoneia (al-ad-zon-i'-a), is an insolent and empty assurance, to trust in ones own power and resources and shamefully despises and violates divine laws and human rights, an impious and empty presumption which trusts in the stability of earthy things.

For all that in the world, the lust of the flesh, and the lust of the eyes, and the pride [212] of life, is not of the Father, but is of the world. **1 John 2:16**

Having pride is to think of our self as higher than we should, to think our ways are better than God's ways, an attitude of "I can do it, I don't need God." This self-righteousness is the attitude that God hates!

When problems arise, self righteousness and pride is an attitude of thinking we can work things out on our own, instead of seeking God in prayer. This can be a hard lesson to learn as God may have to show you how much (more) we can mess things up by trying to fix things on our own.

Do you take credit for your own accomplishments and ideas instead of giving the credit to God? All good things come from God (and have little to do with us) *..to every man that is among you, not to think [of himself] more highly than he ought to think; but to think soberly...* **Romans 12:3**

Taking credit for what God has done for us is very prideful. God hates pride so much that He warns us that He will *bring thee down from thence*, if necessary. Having God humble us, is not a pleasant experience. He would much rather we humble ourselves. And if you have ever been humbled by God, you can testify with me that it is much better to humble yourself.

Thy terribleness hath deceived thee, and the pride of thine heart, O thou that dwellest in the clefts of the rock, that holdest the height of the hill: though thou shouldest make thy nest as high as the eagle, I will bring thee down from thence, saith the LORD. **Jeremiah 49:16**

Do we all need humbling? Apparently so, the prophet Jeremiah tells us: *The heart is deceitful above all things, and desperately wicked: who can know it?* **Jeremiah 17:9**

We are blinded to our sinfulness, but God sees and is able to inspect the true sinfulness of our hearts. It is folly to trust in man, for he is weak, false and deceitful. Our own hearts (because we are human) and emotions deceive us as much as anything. We think that we trust in God when really we do not. If we truly had our trust in God, we would not get nervous, upset, fearful or even react in any way when there is a sudden downturn of our circumstances. There is no reason to fear, there is no reason to worry (if you are truly trusting in God).

The reaction of the people to the terrorist attacks September 11, 2001, and the threat of more or of war, clearly demonstrates that we (as a nation) are not putting our trust where we should. Panic and fear swept through the country and world as if we had no God whatsoever! People were afraid to fly, afraid to leave their homes, afraid to drink the water, open their mail, etc.

Who (or what) do we really depend upon in a day of

9

distress? Do you think that man in the glory of his own wisdom can outwit or evade the enemy? A man's wisdom may fail him when he needs it most, and he may be taken in his own craftiness. To trust in anything other than God is pure foolishness! (And even worse, can turn into idolatry.)

The fact that we are now aware of or even suspect the existence of this wickedness in our hearts is a common mistake. We often think ourselves, our own hearts at least, better than we really are. We often don't acknowledge that our impure thoughts, motives, lusts, bitterness, judging and criticism of others, even if it is not spoken out loud, is sinful in God's eyes. Yet, it is so easy to spot the faults and sin in another.

The heart, the conscience of man, in his corrupt and fallen state, is deceitful above all things. It is subtle and false. It cheats men into their own ruin; and this will be the aggravation of it, that they are self-deceivers, self-destroyers. This is why the heart is desperately wicked.

The heart is so deceitful the Word says, *Who can know it?* Who can describe how bad the heart really is? This reveals we <u>cannot even know our own hearts</u>. We do not know what we (or someone else) will do in an hour of temptation (Hezekiah did not, Peter did not). It tells us we cannot understand our own errors, much less can we know the hearts of others, or have any dependence upon them.

But, whatever wickedness there is in the heart, **God sees it,** and knows it; *I the Lord search the heart.* He knows our thoughts, those that are carelessly overlooked by ourselves. He knows our true intentions. He

10

also clearly tells us not to trust others. *It is better to trust in the LORD than to put confidence in man.* **Psalm 118:8** *Put not your trust in princes, nor in the son of man, in whom there is no help.* **Psalm 146:3**

This is why God is Judge himself, and He alone knows the hearts of men. God observes and discerns them; and (which is more than any man can do) He judges the heart. God knows more evil of us than we do of ourselves, which is a good reason why we should not flatter ourselves, but always stand in awe and fear of the judgment of God.

Humility

Humility is the opposite of pride. Fasting is a tremendous humbling experience. It reveals how weak we really are. It reveals our humanness. Many times in the scriptures, God tells us to humble ourselves.

Humble yourselves therefore under the mighty hand of God, that he may exalt you in due time. **1 Peter 5:6**

For thus saith the high and lofty One that inhabiteth eternity, whose name is Holy; I dwell in the high and holy place, with him also that is of a contrite and humble spirit, to revive the spirit of the humble, and to revive the heart of the contrite ones. **Isaiah 57:15**

Humility and Attitude

Everyone who exalts himself will be abased, and he who humbles himself will be exalted. **Luke 18:13-14**

When we humble ourself to God we can then enter into new realms of obedience, godly growth, and service. While God is always growing us up, we can NEVER think we have arrived!

In Matthew 6:16-18, fasting is described by Jesus as a duty required of disciples of Christ as a means to dispose (prepare) us for other duties. Fasting is a humbling of the soul. *But as for me, when they were sick, my clothing was sackcloth: I humbled my soul with fasting; and my prayer returned into mine own bosom.* **Psalm 35:13**

Jesus tells us that fasting should not be for show (for others). He tells us to fast *unto thy Father which is in secret: and thy Father, which seeth in secret, shall reward thee openly.* **Matthew 6:18**

In all (works) we do, we should have the right motive doing things for God not so other's will see what we are doing and take the glory that belongs to God. If other's take notice and give you the praise, then you will have already received your reward and God cannot reward you. Also remember, we do not do things BECAUSE of the reward, but we do things out of obedience and love for God and simply to serve our fellowman.

If you have the wrong attitude, serving can be a miserable and lonely place. Satan will try to steal our joy of serving God and try to make us feel sorry for ourself. Don't let him do this. <u>God will reward all you do when your heart is pure.</u> If someone does notice what you are doing, simply give the glory to God.

We serve (and give) not to receive our reward, but because of our love for God and our desire to please Him. **When** we get to this point, God can truly use us. He knows we will give the glory to Him. He can trust us.

Lukewarm...
Are We Really Operating at 100%?

Fasting reveals the things in our life that are displeasing to God. It shows us our weak areas, the areas that are lukewarm...*So then because thou art lukewarm, and neither cold nor hot, I will spew thee out of my mouth.* **Revelation 3:16**

There have been several interpretations of this verse and what hot and cold mean. This is how God explained it to me; Being lukewarm is neither hot or cold. *For me* or *against me* is the way God sees it. If you are not 100% for Him, then you are against Him. There is no grading curve with God, He will not even accept 99%. God instructs us to give our ALL to Him. That ALL we do should be focused upon Him. He wants our entire life to be about Him, and not ourselves. All means all, nothing less.

*And when **all things** shall be subdued unto him, then shall the Son also himself be subject unto him that put all things under him, that God may be all in all.* **1 Corinthians 15:28**

*For to this end also did I write, that I might know the proof of you, whether ye be obedient in **all things**.* **2 Corinthians 2:9**

Commit thy works *unto the LORD, and thy thoughts shall be established.* **Proverbs 16:3**

13

Wherefore let them that suffer according to the will of God **commit the keeping of their souls** *to Him in well doing, as unto a faithful Creator.* **1 Peter 4:19**

Cast **all** *your anxiety on Him because he cares for you.* **I Peter 5:7** (Focusing on your circumstances is not focusing your ALL upon Him!)

And whatsoever ye do in word or deed, do **all** *in the name of the Lord Jesus, giving thanks to God and the Father by him.* **Colossians 3:17**

These are powerful scriptures, not only for us to meditate on, but to put into practice. We cannot give 99%; 99% is not ALL. ALL means ALL. We cannot do things (works) for the wrong reasons, we must have pure motives. *Thus saith the LORD of hosts; Consider your ways* (**Haggai 1:7**). We cannot volunteer to help on a committee and then grumble and complain about it. We cannot fret and get anxious over our circumstances – no matter what. Do you think that God does not know your son is in prison or that you have cancer or that you are in debt, or that your husband died and left you with four kids or that your husband is not saved and treats your children poorly or that your son-in-law is an alcoholic? Do you think that complaining to your friends or pastor about it everyday is going to help your situation more than what God could do? Sometimes God will just let a situation get worse and worse until we **completely** turn it over to HIM. We must quit worrying and let Him handle it. This also means to be obedient to His instruction.

14

Sure, we pray about it. Sure, it's not easy. Sure, it still hurts. If we do not commit our ALL to Him. Everything, our whole life, our family, our work, our finances, our health, our ALL - then we are not committed 100% (because we are trying to fix things without God), and that means we are, yep... lukewarm.

I know thy works, that thou art neither cold nor hot: I would thou wert cold or hot. So then because thou art lukewarm, and neither cold nor hot, I will spew thee out of my mouth. Because thou sayest, I am rich, and increased with goods, and have need of nothing; and knowest not that thou art wretched, and miserable, and poor, and blind, and naked: I counsel thee to buy of me gold tried in the fire, that thou mayest be rich; and white raiment, that thou mayest be clothed, and that the shame of thy nakedness do not appear; and anoint thine eyes with eyesalve, that thou mayest see. As many as I love, I rebuke and chasten: be zealous therefore, and repent. **Revelation 3:15-19**

If you are not 100% for Him, then you are against Him.

Why God Hates the Lukewarm

Lukewarm is a false representation of hot. You think your coffee is going to be hot, and you take a drink and find it is only lukewarm, yuk! Lukewarm is what you get with hot with cold mixed in. This is like professing to be a Christian, but keeping a leg or arm dangling over the fence in the world. The unsaved and the young Christians see this "lukewarm" behavior and it is confusing and turns them off. They say, "This guy says he is a Christian, but he swears like crazy!" This person says he is a Christian, he goes to church, but he beats his wife and gambles. They say they are Christians, but I saw them going to that raunchy R-rated movie. They say they are Christians, but they are buried in credit card debt. She claims to be a Christian, but gossips about others in the church." This is exactly what God hates!

God gives me lots of "woods" analogies, as I love to spend time hanging out in the woods surrounding my home in Minnesota. One day God showed me that being lukewarm is like a dead tree that falls in the woods. When a tree falls, especially if it is good sized, before it hits the ground, several perfectly healthy, younger trees often get caught up in the branches of the dead tree and get pushed to the ground. They will stay there trapped under the dead tree and probably die if no one comes and frees them.

A falling dead tree can also wound larger mature trees that are nearby. Sometimes a large limb can get broken off. The wounded tree will probably still survive, but it will never be the same.

God does not want younger, less mature Christians to be negatively influenced and pushed down to the ground by dead lukewarm Christians. If no one comes to save them, they may die. Lukewarm (hypocritical) Christians can lure younger Christians into sin as older Christians serve as mentors and examples for the younger. The penalty for leading younger Christians astray is severe. Jesus said, *And whosoever shall*

offend one of these little ones that believe in me, it is bet-
ter for him that a millstone were hanged about his neck,
and he were cast into the sea. **Mark 9:42**

You may not realize that your actions and words (contradictory to what you profess your faith is or to God) are noticed by others but indeed they are. Our faults are often more quickly noticed by others than we realize them ourselves.

God also wants to prevent other mature Christians from getting wounded as a result of another falling. but it does happen. It is especially painful to be wounded by a brother or sister in Christ. Such woundings often cause people to leave the church. While some may change to another church, others may give up on all Christians and God all together.

Lukewarm is professing to be a Christian, but keeping a leg or arm dangling over the fence in the world.

We are warned of the seriousness of lukewarmness or indifference in our faith. If our faith is real, it is an awesome thing. If it is not real (not 100%), it is repulsive to God, and we should be against it. If our faith is worth anything, it is worth everything; an indifference here is inexcusable.

Can we really be 100%? I don't know, but I know it should be our goal. We do need to realize the areas in our life that are holding us back. The word says we can do all things through Christ who strengthens us.

We not feel condemned just because we are not as mature in our walk or relationship with Him than someone else. God sees our heart and attitude. If pride tells us that we are perfect, God hates that. If we humbly strive to be more like God, He will honor that. God is interested in the purity of our hearts and He knows more than us if that is the case. *He that hath clean hands, and a pure heart; who hath not lifted up his soul unto vanity, nor sworn deceitfully.* Psalms 24:4

Christ expects that we should declare ourselves *"With me"* or *"against me."* (Matthew 12:30) If we are not 100% *with him*, the punishment is severe: *I will spew thee out of my mouth.* The word spew means *to vomit*, or *to cast out with force*. Lukewarm Christians turn the heart of Christ against them. He is greatly grieved by them, and cannot long bear them. Those who are lukewarm (in most all situations), will not know it. Irregardless, it is nauseous to Christ, and they shall be rejected, and finally rejected; for Jesus will not return to that which has been rejected. Once you are rejected, there is no chance of return. Like getting caught up in the force of a powerful river off a cliff, one cannot save themselves and will be cast off the edge, forced out, with no chance for return.

This reminds me of the water that Satan spewed out of his mouth in attempts to overtake the woman in Revelation. *And the serpent cast out of his mouth water as a flood after the woman, that he might cause her to be carried away of the flood.* **Revelation 12:15**

This story clearly reveals the enraged fury of Satan in his desire to destroy Christians. *And the earth* helped the woman, and the earth opened her mouth, and swallowed up the flood which the dragon cast out of his mouth. And the dragon was wroth with the woman, and went to make war with the remnant of her seed, which keep the commandments of God, and have the testimony of Jesus Christ. **Revelation 12:16-17**

We need to take this scripture very seriously. Satan has waged war on all Christians. He is not so concerned about the rest of the world as they are already in the palm of his hand. His attack is specifically directed at those whose name has been written in the Lamb's Book of Life since the beginning.

I strongly believe God is calling His children to WAKE UP! Wake up out of the dangerous dabbling in the world. We simply cannot have one foot in the world thinking it is no big deal (to continue to hold onto a few worldly practices) and assume we are saved Christians. This is lukewarm behavior and **God will not stand for it.** The world is a pagan system. The prince of the world is Satan.

Now is the judgment of this world: now shall the prince of this world be cast out. **John 12:31**

The Blind Leading the Blind

We need to realize that we are indeed blinded by Satan and the ways he pulls us into the world without our knowledge. We need to realize HOW we are being deceived by the world so that we can repent and back out or, even better, avoid it completely.

The main problem is that because most people are blinded, they cannot and do not see the problem. We

19

do not see the trap. We need to pray (all of us) that God removes the scales from our eyes so we can see what we have been blinded to - how we have been deceived. We also need to be prepared to start cleaning up our act, and if God says something has, "Gotta go," then to be obedient and repent from that behavior.

I hear over and over from people, "I am a good Christian. I lead a good life, what's wrong with _____?" (fill in the worldly behavior). For each person it is different.

For me, God has been dealing with these things one by one. Many years ago I was convicted against fast food, convenience foods, junk food, pop, reliance upon pharmaceuticals and the corrupt medical and insurance industries.

Then, I was convicted against secular music and television. Now I wonder how could anyone who calls themself a Christian watch some of these talk-shows which display vile and vulgar Sodom and Gomorah-behavior of people, as if it were something to be proud of and as entertainment? (The Bible says not to even speak of such behavior!) This is reckless and irresponsible desensitization of immoral behavior to the population. The same applies to daytime drama (soap-operas), sitcoms, romance novels, and the list goes on and on.

Things of vanity (cosmetic surgery, artificial nails, jewelry, etc.) are also something we need to be very careful with. I understand that women want to look their best and so wear makeup and have their hair colored, etc. To an extent, this is actually Biblical; *For after this manner in the old time the holy women also,* who trusted in God, adorned themselves (to beautify themselves), being in subjection unto their own husbands, **1 Peter 3:5.** It is important to look the best you can: *Let thy garments be always white; and let thy head lack no ointment,* **Ecclesiastes 9:8,** as long as it does not cross the line into vanity, pride and to show off. *In like manner also, that women adorn themselves in modest apparel, with shamefacedness and sobriety; not with braided hair, or gold, or pearls, or costly array,* **1 Timothy 2:9.**

There is a fine line between enhancing the assets that God blessed you with, versus changing your appearance completely for the sake of vanity. Excess makeup, colored contact lenses, multiple surgical procedures, etc. can completely change a person's appearance. It concerns me if without makeup people don't recognize you because you look so different. I realize this is a sensitive area for many women. If you seek God and you do not feel convicted, then you have nothing to worry about!

Beauty pageants, for example... I cannot imagine that Jesus would think these are a good idea. How is parading around in a bathing suit complete with breast and rear enhancers, in high heels NOT degrading to women?

The world would also have us all believe that we all need some sort of psychiatric therapy to get along in the world; group therapy, self-help groups, self-help books, Alcoholics Anonymous, Al-Anon, and on and on. People will spend thousands and thousands of dollars for counseling (of a non-Christian nature) of some sort or another. How sad that we are not reaching out to others and that people actually have to pay someone to listen to them, or to counsel married couples how to get along when the Bible gives us all the instruction we need.

For all our "problems" there is only one solution: JESUS! He already paid the price for us in full and we don't need to spend a dime more! We need to repent from our sins, lay our burdens at the feet of Jesus, and break off the yoke of guilt and shame and condemnation!

We also need to know who we are doing business with. We cannot assume that all businesses are run ethically or even legally. Practice discernment. Don't enter into business deals with just anyone; you may end up with Satan as your business partner! Much of the business world would not survive if Christians would quit supporting the one's with questionable ethics, products and etc. We need to stop going along with what everyone else is doing and what everyone else is buying.

The entertainment industry would also have a hard time staying in business if Christians quit purchasing, attending and renting all the immoral materials produced today. Maybe it would at least influence them to produce more wholesome entertainment.

Commercialism (advertising and marketing) is a huge business, and it is all about manipulation. The sole purpose of advertising and marketing in the world is to convince you that you need to buy something that you do not need. If you needed it, you would probably buy it and therefore you do not need the advertisement. Every possible angle has been used, and companies are continually looking for more ways to entice you to buy what they want you to; for sake of convenience, taste, sympathy, ego, pride, vanity, or just because it is a good bargain. Have you ever bought something just because it was on sale? Or justified a purchase in your mind because it was on sale?

How many times do you run into the store to get one or two things and end up buying a whole bunch of extra stuff that you didn't know you *needed* till you saw it? For those in advertising and marketing: mission accomplished.

There is every imaginable scheme and scam out there: Plans for you to get rich, to get out of debt, to work at home and get rich, to lose weight, to have perfect skin, to grow hair, to improve your sex life, to provide you with a sex life, to send you on vacation for "free," that will only cost you..., to increase your business sales, to save you money (how does *spending* money on what they are selling you *save* you money?) and on and on. You would save more money, by *not buying* into what they are selling you. We are all tired of the soliciting phone calls and junk mail, but there are a lot more subtle schemes that we do not recognize as such.

I know a dental hygienist who was employed at a certain dental office with several dentists. She was fired because she did not meet their "standards of productivity." Meaning, each hygienist was expected to direct a certain percentage of their patients for more extensive periodontal work done (to bring in more revenue for the business). It was the practice of the business to have the hygienist even use "scare tactics" on the patients so they would have additional more expensive treatments done - <u>whether they needed it or not.</u>

Many cases of gum inflammation will easily be remedied by the routine cleaning the hygienist is supposed to be doing so that further work will not be needed at all. But instead, the patient may be warned about the seriousness of periodontal disease and told that an extensive $1,600 scaling is available, which would take care of the problem. However, if the patient did not have insurance, they could *try* to do lesser invasive scaling for only $400.00.

These questionable (to put it mildly) tactics are commonly used not only in the dental industry, but the whole medical industry and the rest of the business world. I have not only witnessed and experienced such behavior in dental and doctor offices, but at the veterinarian, the auto mechanic, the beauty salon, and many other places. As this is more common in metropolitan areas; there is something good to be said for small, reliable "hometown" practices.

Because this particular moral and ethical dental hygienist would not "sell" procedures to patients that did not need them, she was fired. This is exactly the kind of commitment God wants from us. What would you do?

She is now thankful that she was fired as she did not want to work at a place that did not have the same standards of ethics that she did.

This is also a good lesson for all of you who are job hunting. Be sure to know the people and the standards of business that an organization operates under before you become involved with them. If you are not careful, they can manipulate you to lower your standards just because you fear losing your job, or for other reasons.

Some companies pay commissions for productivity of their employees. This can be a dangerous trap. *For the love of money is the root of all evil: which while some coveted after, they have erred from the faith, and pierced themselves through with many sorrows.* **1 Timothy 6:10**

We Deceive Ourselves

Self-delusion (we convince ourselves that what is untrue or is not of God, is true, or we deny that what *is* true and from God) is among the greatest problems for Christians. You may call it legalism, a spirit of religion, a spirit of deceit or a lying spirit. You may call it pride. Whatever you call it, it is very dangerous. As long as you allow it to remain - it will. By NOT commanding it and sincerely wanting it to depart from you, you are giving it permission to stay. To do this you have to admit that it is present. Because of the nature of the spirit, this is the largest part of the battle. You may think, "I have no sin, what am I doing wrong?" You may justify your thoughts or actions, while inwardly condemning others for theirs.

As those who think they are well enough already (don't need God), therefore, can be very indifferent to whether they grow (better, closer to Him) or not. If you do not truly believe, *I am blessed and have need of nothing,* financial and physical needs can cause one to overlook the necessities of their souls. One who thinks he is rich may be actually very poor if they have no provision for their souls. One who thinks themself spiritually sound (because they attend church, tithe, pray, don't curse, etc.), can be deceived in the name of religion.

Christ counsels us to drop a vain and false opinion

we may have of ourselves: *I counsel thee to buy of me,* etc. Even though these people were poor; Christ counsels them to <u>buy of him</u> gold tried in the fire, that they might be rich. To do this, something (other than money) must be parted with; this is to "make room" to receive His true riches. *Part with sin and self-sufficiency, and come to Christ with a sense of your poverty and emptiness, that you may be filled with his hidden treasure.*

Those who are blind cannot see their true state, nor realize the danger they are in. The blind cannot comprehend all what Christ has done for them. If they get a promotion in their job, they think is it because of their own hard work. If they are able to buy a new car at a greatly reduced price, they think they are lucky or that they are shrewd in negotiations. The blind are counseled to buy of him eye-salve, that they might see, to give up their own wisdom and reason.

Christ tells the naked they might have clothing, and such as would cover the shame of their nakedness. For this they must receive from Christ; and they must only put off their filthy rags (give up and turn from their sin) that they might put on the white raiment which He had purchased and provided for them—His own imputed righteousness for justification and the garments of holiness and sanctification.

They were without God, and He has been the dwelling-place of His people in all ages; in Him alone the soul of man can find rest, and safety, and all suitable accommodations. The riches of the body and the world will not enrich the soul; the sight of the body will not enlighten the soul; the most convenient house for the body will not afford rest nor safety to the soul. No matter how the body may seem to be prospering, the soul can be wretched and miserable.

After all of this, He warns the lukewarm they will be spewed out... *As many as I love, I rebuke and chasten: be zealous therefore, and repent. Behold, I stand at the door, and knock: if any man hear my voice, and open the door, I will come in to him, and will sup with him, and he with me.* **Revelation 3:19-20**

If God did not love us, He would have no reason to rebuke and chasten us. He would ignore our sinful lukewarmness and vain confidence if He hated us. He would have simply let us alone, to go on in sin until it had been our ruin. It is the nature of sin to cause pain and destroy.

The Stuff That's "Gotta Go!"

Fasting is about training your mind to focus on God. It is a time of self-examination and realization of how weak we are. We need to train ourselves to resist the world every day... to put Jesus and His desire for our life above all else.

Part of the power and significance of fasting is that in growing closer to God, He starts revealing some of the things that He requires us to get rid of. Things that are not all necessarily sin, but things which are interfering with a perfect relationship with Him, the Holy one.

Let us search and try our ways, and turn again to the LORD. Lamentations 3:40

1. Self

The **"Death to Self"** issue is one of the most difficult things we need to learn as Christians. Self is the flesh and all of our fleshly desires that we must give up. It is what we want. It is what (we think) makes us feel good. It is what (we think) will satisfy our needs and longings. We must "die" to the flesh.

For if ye live after the flesh, ye shall die: but if ye through the Spirit do mortify the deeds of the body, ye shall live. **Romans 8:13**

The bottom line is a difficult lesson to learn: **"We can't always have what we want…. or when we want it."** Just because we want it doesn't mean it is good for us. If it is not something that God grants you, it does not mean it is bad either. Sometimes God just says "No" as if to remind us of who is in control. God may have something better in mind… or is showing us that you just need to wait. God's timing is perfect. The waiting, of course, is another very difficult concept for us to grasp. We grow tired and impatient and start thinking of things we could do (on our own) to rectify the situation.

As we grow in our relationship with God, we can look back at all the times that we didn't wait for God - where we took matters into our own hands (often referred to as running ahead of God) and really messed things up for ourselves. After doing this a few times, we see how important it is just to wait… but, that doesn't make the waiting any easier. (And don't complain about the waiting either. The Israelites ended up in the desert 40 years because of their complaining and murmuring!)

I do not understand what I do, for what I want to

*do I do not do and want I hate to do, that do I. As it is,
it is no longer I myself who do it, but it is sin living in me.
I know that nothing good lives in me, that is, in my sinful nature.* **Romans 7:15, 17-18** NIV

We must put aside (or put into perspective) what
we want (desires of the flesh and the desires of our
heart) and concentrate on what God wants for us and
what He wants us to be doing. THEN, He will be able to
bless us with what He knows is best for us – in His
perfect timing. Whether it be a helpmate, children, a
new house, car or other material or financial needs.
God will provide all of our needs, including the desires
of our heart. **(Psalm 37: 3-7)**

Some things are very difficult to wait for: pregnan-
cy if you and your spouse are trying to have children; a
spouse for those who are single or widowed; healing in
the case of a serious illness or pain; freedom from debt,
a job; a son, daughter or spouse to be delivered from
drug or alcohol addiction or from some other bondage in
their life. We want to rescue them, we can't stand to see
them suffer, but there are some things we cannot do for
other people, we wait for God and pray.

Many times, as we wait, God wants us to be working on ourselves, He wants us to grow in our faith and
in our trust in Him that He will take care of us and will
do a much better job than we can do ourselves.

*The righteous cry, and the LORD heareth, and deliv-
ereth them out of all their troubles. The LORD is nigh
unto them that are of a broken heart; and saveth such
as be of a contrite spirit. Many are the afflictions of the
righteous: but the LORD delivereth him out of them all.*

The LORD redeemeth the soul of his servants: and none of them that trust in him shall be desolate. **Psalm 34:17-19, 22**

The eyes of all wait upon thee; and thou givest them their meat in due season. **Psalm 145:15**

And therefore will the LORD wait, that he may be gracious unto you, and therefore will he be exalted, that he may have mercy upon you: for the LORD is a God of judgment: blessed are all they that wait for him. **Isaiah 30:18**

But they that wait upon the LORD shall renew their strength; they shall mount up with wings as eagles; they shall run, and not be weary; and they shall walk, and not faint. **Isaiah 40:31**

2. Faith in Man and the World

In Paul's letter to the Colossians he warns them of the traps of the world. He warns them if they get caught up in the world that they will become dead to Christ. This is very serious. If we are numb to the prompting of the Holy Spirit, what guide will we have to lead us? How will we know if involvement in this or that is acceptable to Him? He is clearly warning us that if we are listening to the world and not the Holy Spirit, we can only get sucked in. These things (of the world) serve only the flesh and not God.

See to it that no one carries you off as spoil or makes you yourselves captive by his so-called philosophy and intellectualism and vain deceit (idle fancies and plain nonsense), following human tradition (man's idea of the material rather than the spiritual world), just crude notions fol-

30

lowing rudimentary and elementary teachings of the universe and disregarding (the teachings of) Christ, the messiah. **Colossians 2:8** AMP

Wherefore if ye be dead with Christ from the rudiments of the world, why, as though living in the world, are ye subject to ordinances, (Touch not; taste not; handle not; Which all are to perish with the using;) after the commandments and doctrines of men? Which things have indeed a shew of wisdom in will worship, and humility, and neglecting of the body; not in any honor to the satisfying of the flesh. **Colossians 2:20-23**

If you have died with Christ to material ways of looking at things, then why do you live as though you still belong in the world? Why do you listen to what other's are saying (other than God)? The world is promoting and indulging the flesh; it does not promote self-control, or any other virtues of God.

Much of the book of Revelation talks about the fall of man; how man is deceived by things like religion, man, wealth, satan and all the things of the world.

This know also, that in the last days perilous times shall come. For men shall be lovers of their own selves, covetous, boasters, proud, blasphemers, disobedient to parents, unthankful, unholy, Without natural affection, trucebreakers, false accusers, incontinent, fierce, despisers of those that are good, Traitors, heady, highminded, lovers of pleasures more than lovers of God; **Having a form of godliness, but denying the power thereof: from such turn away.** *For of this sort are they which creep into houses, and lead captive silly* *women laden with sins, led away with divers lusts, Ever learning, and never able to come to the knowledge of the truth.* **2 Timothy 3:1-7**

This is quite a list. At first it may seem like a list of godless sinners in the world. But take close notice that these individuals who "appear to be godly" are grouped among those who covet, boast, have pride, are unholy, liars, and etc. We are not talking about the unsaved. We are talking about those in the church, whose salvation (unknowst) to them is in question.

The perilous times in the last days that Paul refers to deal with **the way** that Satan will (is now) deceiving us. He is alerting us to those who "have a form of godliness" who shall be corrupt and wicked, and do a great deal of damage in the church.

From these things, Christians must withdraw themselves. Although the times may seem chaotic, God has it all under His control. Satan can deceive the nations and the churches no further and no longer than God will permi. Satan and those under his lead shall be exposed, and every man shall abandon them.

Mark of the Beast: 666

And that no man might buy or sell, save he that had the mark, or the name of the beast, or the number of his name. Here is wisdom. Let him that hath understanding count the number of the beast: for it is the number of a man; and his number is 666. **Revelation 13:17-18**

666 is the number of the beast, given in such a manner as shows the infinite wisdom of God, and will sufficiently exercise all the wisdom and accuracy of

men: The number 6 is the number of a man.

666 is *man, man, man,* which replaces the Holy trinity: Father, Son and Holy Ghost. This revelation is very clear to me. God is telling us: Do not allow man to replace the Father. Do not allow man to replace the Son. Do not allow man to replace the Holy Spirit.

Do not forget, we are dealing with the DECEIVER. He has been deceiving the world since the beginning and is very good at it. No one (except Christ) is above the deceit and tricks of Satan. If you think that Satan cannot trick you, you have already been tricked.

Let no man deceive himself. If any man among you seemeth to be wise in this world, let him become a fool, that he may be wise. **1 Corinthians 3:18**

Satan comes in the form and shape of a lamb (the angel of light). Under the pretense of religion, he deceives the souls of men with false doctrines and cruel decrees which show him to belong to the dragon, and not to the Lamb.

This is cause for great alarm, because we are not talking about people in the world (non-Christians) being deceived, but people in the church.

And the first went, and poured out his vial upon the earth; and there fell a noisome and grievous sore upon the men which had the mark of the beast, and upon them which worshiped his image. **Revelation 16:2**

And the beast was taken, and with him the false prophet that wrought miracles before him, with which he deceived them that had received the mark of the beast, and them that worshiped his image. These both were cast alive into a lake of fire burning with brimstone.

33

Revelation 19:20

We must realize the very important concept that "his image" is **anything** of the World. Satan has deceived us with traps like wealth, success, power, material goods ("things"), relationships, food, medicine, pharmaceuticals, drugs and alcohol, sex, pornography, credit cards, youthfulness and physical attractiveness, and the list goes on and on.

Commercialism and consumerism in the prosperous Western nations literally has us all fooled into thinking that we need all sorts of "things" for one reason or another. We are convinced it is more important to "have" (what we think we want or need) than it is to be godly, and to be a person of integrity, respect, honor, temperance, peace, love and joy.

Love not the world, neither the things that are in the world. If any man love the world, the love of the Father is not in him. **1 John 2:15**

Wealth and riches is one of the biggest stumbling blocks to our faith in God. When many people think of "sinners" they only think of the poor, the "down and outers," but I suspect that a much greater number of individuals are those who have so much wealth that in their own minds, because they have all they need, and then some, are perfectly content, having an attitude, "What do I need that religion stuff for?" Not having a clue even of what they are missing out on. They don't realize how unhappy they really are, living without true peace and joy in their life.

Even those considered "middle class" can get

caught up in this false thinking. "We have all we need, we're not into church, they just want to take your money anyway." There's no time (made) for God (or church) with both parents working and taking the kids to this and that. Their needs seem to be met (superficially) so they don't even recognize the significance of their need for Christ. They don't see their own selfish attitudes.

They shall cast their silver in the streets, and their gold shall be removed: their silver and their gold shall not be able to deliver them in the day of the wrath of the LORD: they shall not satisfy their souls, neither fill their bowels: because **it (wealth) is the stumbling block of their iniquity. Ezekiel 7:19**

It is the intention of Satan to fool us into thinking that we do not need God. He preys on our weaknesses, our fleshly desires to be successful and prosperous. He preys on our desires to provide for our loved ones, thinking they will love us more if we can afford to buy them anything they want. We confuse the issues of gift giving and love.

For we wrestle not against flesh and blood, but against principalities, against powers, against the rulers of the darkness of this world, against spiritual wickedness in high places. **Ephesians 6:12**

Another trap Satan has set for us is all the systems of the world. These are things that God does not require of us, but the world tries to convince us that we must do or we must have. Note that these things ultimately or directly result in the financial gain of someone. Examples are: Life insurance, medical insurance, dental insurance, vaccinations, etc. Car insurance is required by law if you drive a car, and therefore, we should obey, but the others are not. They use fear to convince us that we "need" these things.

Credit cards, bank cards, and companies who want to set up automatic transfers from your bank account for bill payments are examples of companies using fear-based manipulation. They try to convince you it is more convenient and sometimes even offer discounts if you allow them to do this.

Consider the cost of a funeral, caskets, burial or cremation, cemetery plots and head stones! Do you really think this is pleasing to God to go to such extravagant lengths and expense to deal with a body no longer containing a spirit or soul? But most people just go along with it, paying the ridiculous prices. Hey, when I am gone, I hope everyone I know is REJOICING because I am finally home with my Lord! This place is not my home, so dig a hole in my woods, throw some leaves over what's left of me and go celebrate! What a waste of money and land to do anything more!

Vaccinations, flu shots, pharmaceuticals, the list goes on and on, don't conform to these things without checking with God first. The world (man, government, etc.) often even tries to force us to do these things. God tells us not to fall for the snares that man has set. If you are falling into these traps (going along with whatever people tell you or the current traditions of the world are) and not seeking the counsel of God or His opinion of these things, then you have been deceived.

The proud have hid a snare for me, and cords; they

have spread a net by the wayside; they have set gins for me. Selah. **Psalm 140:5**

Wherefore I also said, I will not drive them out from before you; but they shall be as thorns in your sides, and their gods shall be a snare unto you. **Judges 2:3**

For man also knoweth not his time: as the fishes that are taken in an evil net, and as the birds that are caught in the snare; so are the sons of men snared in an evil time, when it falleth suddenly upon them. **Ecclesiastes 9:12**

So, you ask, how are we replacing God (Father, Son and Holy Ghost) with man (and the world)? The sad truth is that we do it all the time. Most of the time, we just do not realize it. If there is a problem with a kitchen appliance, what do you do first? Get out the manual, call a repair person, call the manufacturer, call your husband, or pray? Sometimes prayer is not even on the list of things we do.

If you had a stressful day at work, what do you do? Call a friend? Look for sympathy and affection from your spouse? Pour a drink? Eat chocolate? Chips? Drink a cola or beer? Go shopping? Go to the refrigerator? Order a pizza? Turn on the TV to veg? Go to the gym? Go running? *(unless you pray when you are running!)*

This is what God is talking about. If we go to anything or anyone other than God, we are really seeking man (or the world) first instead of Him. We are to seek God first for all of our needs.

I will cry unto God most high; unto God that performeth all things for me. **Psalm 57:2**

.37

Cast thy burden upon the LORD, and he shall sustain thee: he shall never suffer the righteous to be moved. **Psalm 55:22**

Whatever it is that thou desire from God, leave it to Him to give it in his own way and time. *Cast thy care upon the Lord.* **1 Peter 5:7**

When our circumstances become difficult, we MUST learn to NOT react out of our emotions. Things like fear, anger, etc., distract us even further, which is exactly what the enemy wants. **(Matthew 6:25; Psalm 84:11; Romans 8:28**.) If we seek God, He will give us the wisdom or comfort that is needed to deal with whatever situation is at hand. We can waste a lot of time, money and energy trying to deal with things on our own.

Whom (or What) Do You Seek?

Who do you seek first when you are feeling down and depressed or when your circumstances take a turn for the worse? A friend? Your spouse? Your kids? Maybe even alcohol or drugs? Go shopping? Do you bury yourself in work (or business)? Or do you just plain bury it, pretending it will go away?

Who do you seek first when you are sick? God or man? We have become (a little too) accustomed to going to the doctor or taking a pill when we are sick. We desire instant results maybe by taking a prescription vs. the nothingness we may often (think that we) hear when we pray for healing or for direction from God. It is not that He is not answering us, sometimes we just don't hear him. We may not want to accept that we need to change our (stinking) thinking, lifestyle or eating habits because that is what got us sick in the first place. God isn't going to heal you when you are living in disobedience and violating your own body. If He does heal you, you cannot expect to hold onto your supernatural blessing by continuing to violate God's natural laws for the body or if you continue to agree with the lie that opened the door for Satan to bring sickness to you.

I had gotten prayer many times for cold sores in the 5 years since I started getting them. Each time I believed I was healed... but would get another. I tried taking Lysine and special creams... nothing helped. FINALLY, I discovered the ROOT of problem. It relates to Diana, the godess of beauty (Artemis) as described in Acts 21, as a spirit of ugly. I was coming into agreement with the LIE (from Satan) that I was not beautiful (which is NOT how God sees me). This is what was opening the door for the attack (making me really ugly). Now that I have repented and asked God to help me see myself as He sees me - because He thinks we are all beautiful, I do believe I am now healed forever! Praise God!

It is very important to search for the root of your health problems. Fasting is an excellent way to do this. We must be in agreement with God and the way He thinks so He can protect us and keep us in divine health!

Whoever is of God heareth God's words. (Those who belong to Him hear the words of God.) This is the reason that you do not listen (to those words, to Me); because you do not belong to God and are not of Him or in harmony with Him. **John 8:47** AMP

When we are sick, instead of going to the church elders to be prayed for, it is common to go to the doctor where you will often get a prescription. If this does not help, you may get another prescription or go to another doctor where you will get yet another prescription. When this does not work (and now you have the added side effects from the medications) you may consult a specialist or another type of doctor. A naturopath or a chiropractor may recommend dietary changes and supplements. You may take the supplements (for a while), but find it too inconvenient to change your diet and so this approach does not work. You go back to the regular doctor who does painful and humiliating tests, and more tests. Finally, he recommends surgery. You decide to have the surgery and they remove something that was God's perfect plan for your body for a specific reason and function. After the surgery, you are still sick, and now have an entire new onslought of health problems because of the organ removal (that they neglected to inform you about prior to the surgery). So now you have thousands of dollars in medical bills, a pile of very confusing insurance papers, and you are worse off than before you started. So, you finally decide to go up for prayer for healing after a church service - and what happens? God heals you at that moment!

You think this does not happen? This has been happening since the days when Jesus walked the earth! And it is still frequently happening today.

This incidence is recorded in all three Gospels. *And a certain woman, which had an issue of blood twelve years, And had suffered many things of many physicians, and had spent all that she had, and was nothing bettered, but rather grew worse, When she had heard of Jesus, came in the press behind, and touched his garment. For she said, If I may touch but his clothes, I shall be whole. And straightway the fountain of her blood was dried up; and she felt in her body that she was healed of that plague.* **Mark 5:25-29**

Several years ago in a medical exam a "suspicious lump" was found and I was directed to return for a follow-up, and another and another. The testing was becoming more invasive and even painful. I was becoming more and more irritated and tired of going to so many appointments. I decided that this whole doctor thing had gotten out of hand and turned the situation over to God.

The clinic started calling and leaving messages that I needed to come in for my test results. After several calls and letters I finally picked up the phone and told them, that I would not be coming in and that I was not interested in my results. This upset the caller and she started lecturing me on the importance of follow-up and how I needed to come back in and that I needed to come back for another biopsy, etc., but I said, "Thank you, but I would rather pray about it" and hung up. They called back many more times leaving messages instructing me to schedule another appointment until I finally picked up the phone and again told the caller that I was not interested in my results. I then informed them that I was also losing my health insurance (which was true) so I couldn't pay for the treatment even if I did have cancer, so I was going to pray about it. I never heard from them again. Interestingly, at that point they apparently lost interest as they learned I would not be able to pay for additional services.

My story is not uncommon. I continually hear about women who have had total hysterectomies or mastectomies, only to discover later that it was completely unnecessary.

I recently met a women who had a pacemaker implanted, but it was not correcting the problem. At this writing, it is now believed that the problems she was experiencing were the result of an iron-deficiency anemia, which could have been easily corrected without surgery, but with simple supplementation and dietary changes.

I know of several people who had their gall bladders removed, but afterwards their pain and other symptoms were still present. The doctors simply shrugged and said, "it must not have been your gall bladder."

This breaks my heart. God put those organs in us for important functions and we simply cannot live as well without them! We need to be checking in with God for these things. He is the great Physician. If we are having health problems, He knows exactly what is wrong with us and how He wants us to correct it. Where do you put your faith? In doctors (men)? or God? I am not saying that all doctors are bad (don't forget, Luke was a physician). I am saying that man is subject to "human error" and in many cases may be influenced by the "medical-insurance scam/system." How do you know? You had better be in prayer about all such situations. Here is another example.

The 21-year-old son of a friend of mine was in a

tragic car accident. There were severe head injuries and he was in a coma for months. The test results convinced the doctors that he would never recover and would essentially be a "vegetable" for the rest of his life. This is what the hospital told the family. The mother, a powerful and dedicated prayer warrior, knew that God was much bigger than that. She knew in her spirit that her son would be just fine and she told the hospital staff exactly that. She even told the local newspaper and they quoted her. After 8 months of extensive rehabilitation and powerful prayer, that young man is out of his coma, he is alert, is able to walk, and I had a perfectly normal conversation with him in church myself when I saw him. Now it has not been easy for this family, but they stood by the all-powerful God they believed in and trusted that He would get them through this difficult time. As God continues to heal and bless that family for their faithfulness, it stands as a powerful testimony for all of us as to what God can do if you don't cave in to what the world says.

In my first book for God, *God Wants You Well*, I chronicle how God healed my asthma so I no longer require the pharmaceuticals which I relied upon daily for over 20 years of my life. Even before I was a born-again Christian, I had always strongly felt that God did not want us to rely upon pharmaceuticals. This is what the Word says about the use of pharmaceuticals.

The word *pharmacy* comes from the Greek words *pharmakeia* and *pharmakeus* defined from Strongs:

Pharmakeia (Greek 5331) {far-mak-i'-ah}: sorcery 2, witchcraft 1; 3

1) the use or the administering of drugs

2) poisoning

3) sorcery, magical arts, often found in connection with idolatry and fostered by it

4) metaphor- the deceptions and seductions of idolatry

Pharmakeus (Greek 5332) {far-mak-yoos'} from pharmakon (a drug, i.e. spell-giving potion); A druggist "pharmacist" or poisoner: sorcerer.

1) one who prepares or uses magical remedies

2) sorcerer

There are several scriptures which use these Greek terms. All clearly describe the use (reliance upon) of these things (pharmaceuticals, drugs) as sin: *Now the works of the flesh are manifest, which are these; Adultery, fornication, uncleanness, lasciviousness, Idolatry,* **witchcraft (Greek 5331)**, *hatred, variance, emulations, wrath, strife, seditions, heresies.* **Galatians 5:19-20**

But the fearful, and unbelieving, and the abominable, and murderers, and whoremongers, and **sorcerers (Greek 5332)**, *and idolaters, and all liars, shall have their part in the lake which burneth with fire and brimstone: which is the second death.* **Revelation 21:8**

God has a better plan. Ezekiel wrote that the leaves of the trees should be used for medicine.

And by the river upon the bank thereof, on this side and on that side, shall grow all trees for meat, whose leaf shall not fade, neither shall the fruit thereof be consumed: it shall bring forth new fruit according to his months, because their waters they issued out of the sanctuary: and the fruit thereof shall be for meat, and the leaf thereof for medicine. **Ezekiel 47:12** (see also

Revelation 22:2)

God designed the physical body with an incredible ability to continually renew and heal itself.

I will praise thee; for I am fearfully and wonderfully made: marvellous are thy works; and that my soul knoweth right well. **Psalm 139:14**

If we cut ourselves, the tissues are able to mend themselves. If we are exposed to a bacteria or virus, the immune system sends white blood cells to identify, kill and dispose of such undesirables (and also potentially cancerous cells, cellular debris, etc.) in the body. We may suffer some symptoms (runny nose, congestion, headache, fever, diarrhea, etc.) while this happens, but if the immune system is healthy, we will recover.

Man has created all sorts of chemical remedies (drugs) to mask these cold and flu symptoms, but they don't help heal the body in any way. In fact, they may slow down the body's ability to heal itself and have many dangerous side effects. One manufacturer of over-the-counter allergy and cold remedies recently withdrew all of their products containing Pheny-lpropanolamine (PPA) which the FDA recently reported to be linked to increased hemorrhagic stroke (bleeding in brain) and seizures. This drug (also found in weight control appetite suppressants) has been available for years.

We have all experienced infection from what is known as the common cold virus – from which you fully recovered. You may have even heard that without treatment of any kind, the symptoms will last somewhere between 4 and 10 days. If you treat yourself with any of the numerous over-the-counter cold medications, your symptoms will still last somewhere between 4 and 10 days. These are not a cure, they simply help (supposedly) reduce some of the symptoms, but they do have side effects.

However, at first sign of a cold symptom, probably millions of people can testify that by supplementing immune-enhancing nutrients such as vitamin C, zinc, colostrum and medicinal mushrooms, that the cold can be completely warded off and that they experience no other cold symptoms.

We know it is always better to solve the root problem (often a weakened immune system) than to mask the symptoms. There are some drugs which are lifesavers. The problem seems to lie in the daily use and reliance on pharmaceutical drugs. One cannot continue on in the lifestyle that created the health problem and expect that the medication is going to correct the problem. It may help (and even be lifesaving) for a while, but your goal should be to correct (repent from) the cause of the problem.

For example, if a diet high in sugar and refined foods resulted in diabetes, you cannot expect to take medication and or insulin, continue your poor dietary habits, and expect to live in health.

You cannot continue a high sugar, high fat diet resulting in elevated cholesterol and triglyceride levels to be corrected by medication alone. You must go to the source of the problem.

God's perfect plan is not really to heal us but to not have us get sick in the first place. There is overwhelming scientific evidence that the body can protect and heal itself more effectively if we take care of the body through proper nutritional support, avoidance of pollutants and toxins, moderate lifestyle, adequate rest, fresh air and physical activity. PREVENTION is God's plan!

I love the story of Jesus raising the young girl from the dead (Mark 5:37-43). He says to her *"Talitha koum!"* which means "little girl arise", and she did and He told them not to let anyone know about this and *"to give her something to eat."* As God does His part in our healing <u>we are also responsible</u> to take care of and feed our bodies properly.

Christian Living is Healthy Living!

Examples of Putting Your Faith in Man (World) - Instead of God.

✦ Thinking that relational things (being married or having children, etc.) are going to make you happy.

✦ Listening to the counsel of your friends and family instead of seeking the will of God.

✦ Asking your spouse and your friends for advice instead of seeking the will of God

✦ To rely upon pharmaceuticals and advice of doctors instead of seeking the will of God.

✦ To rely upon finances (job, career, etc.) and material things to provide all you need and make you happy.

✦ Seeking horoscope or psychic predictions to give you direction or hope.

✦ Seeking other things for comfort such as food, alcohol, sex, clothes, "toys," etc.

✦ Getting caught up in religious traditions instead of the will of God. Man's traditions interfere with our ability to hear God (mostly because we don't even ask God what His will is in those situations- worldly holiday practices, such as Christmas trees, Easter decorations such as bunnies and eggs (which have their origination in sex and fertility gods.)

God Wants our WHOLE Heart, Mind and Body! What is 100%?

What if God told you to leave your current job, sell your house and move your family to another state? *(How long would it take you to be obedient? Until God makes arrangements for you to be fired?)*

What if God told you to stop tithing at your current church and put your money elsewhere? *(Would you worry about what the people in your church thought?)*

What if God told you to take in someone (of questionable character) who was down and out and just let them stay at your house? *(Would you trust God that He would protect you if you let them stay, or would you*

48

watch them like a hawk and never leave them alone in the house?)

What if God told you to give someone in need your car or a large sum of money? *(Would you expect it back? Would you give them the amount you thought you could afford or the amount that God told you to give?)*

What if God wanted you to quit your job or present work and go into full time ministry? *(Would you put if off until God gave you no choice through the loss of your job or company?)*

What if God wanted you to sell <u>all</u> your possessions, give the money to the poor and follow Him?

And when he was gone forth into the way, there came one running, and kneeled to him, and asked him, Good Master, what shall I do that I may inherit eternal life? And Jesus said unto him, Why callest thou me good? there is none good but one, that is, God. Thou knowest the commandments, Do not commit adultery, Do not kill, Do not steal, Do not bear false witness, Defraud not, Honor thy father and mother. And he answered and said unto him, Master, all these have I observed from my youth.

Then Jesus beholding him loved him, and said unto him, One thing thou lackest: go thy way, sell whatsoever thou hast, and give to the poor, and thou shalt have treasure in heaven: and come, take up the cross, and follow me. And he was sad at that saying, and went away grieved: for he had great possessions.

And Jesus looked round about, and saith unto his disciples, How hardly shall they that have riches enter into the kingdom of God! And the disciples were astonished at his words. But Jesus answereth again, and saith unto them, Children, how hard is it for them that trust in riches to enter into the kingdom of God! It is easier for a camel to go through the eye of a needle, than for a rich man to enter into the kingdom of God. **Mark 10:17-25**

Note: The eye of a needle is said to be a rock formation in Israel. It is a very narrow passageway, much like the eye of a needle. In order to go through, a camel, which carries all of the belongings of a person, must remove all of its baggage.

The Deceit

No one likes getting lied to. No one likes to be deceived, AND I think probably the worst part about deceit, is that the one being deceived, DOES NOT KNOW IT!

And the light of a candle shall shine no more at all in thee; and the voice of the bridegroom and of the bride shall be heard no more at all in thee: for thy merchants were the great men of the earth; for by thy sorceries were all nations deceived. **Revelation 18:23**

Revelation Chapter 18 discusses the downfall of Babylon (representing the world). An angel proclaims the fall of Babylon assigning the reasons of her fall. She gives warning to all who belonged to God to come out of her, and to assist in her destruction. Great lamentation were made for her by those who had been large sharers in her sinful pleasures and profits. Babylon's friends are the mourners, namely, those who had been bewitched by her fornication, those who had been sharers in her sensual pleasures, and those who had been gainers by her wealth and trade—the kings and the merchants of the earth; the kings of the earth, whom she had flattered into idolatry by allowing them to be arbitrary and tyrannical over those under them (employees, etc.); and the merchants, that is, those who trafficked with her for indulgences, pardons, dispensations, and preferments; these will mourn, because by this craft they got their wealth. They mourn not because of their sin, but because of their great losses.

We Deceive Ourselves

If it were not bad enough that the world (continually and constantly) deceives us, sometimes our biggest enemy can be our own self. We think, *"well, I'm not so bad. I'm not like those people* (who we PERCEIVE to be the sinners). *I don't do this or that like those people do."* Paul can quickly put us in our place: *As it is written, There is none righteous, no, not one: There is none that understandeth, there is none that seeketh after God.* **Romans 3:10-11**

God is not just concerned about sin that other people see, He is concerned about the things that only He sees - like your thoughts or motives!

For all have sinned, and come short of the glory of God. **Romans 3:23** Thank goodness Paul follows this statement with: *All are justified and made upright and in right standing with God, freely and gratuitously by His*

51

grace (His unmerited favor and mercy), through the redemption which is (provided) in Christ Jesus. **Romans 3:23** AMP

One of the reasons that fasting is so important and so humbling is that God reveals much of what sin there is in our life that we may be denying (hiding, burying, etc.). Big sin, little sin, it's all the same to Him. I tell God, *"I'm a bad faster (because I am so weak), why am I writing this book?"* He just says, *"That's why."* God will still use us for His purpose just as we are. *But God hath chosen the foolish things of the world to confound the wise; and God hath chosen the weak things of the world to confound the things which are mighty.* **1 Corinthians 1:27**

Therefore I take pleasure in infirmities, in reproaches, in necessities, in persecutions, in distresses for Christ's sake: for when I am weak, then am I strong. **2 Corinthians 12:10**

3. Guilt, Shame, Condemnation

People hate to feel guilty. Many would much rather either justify the actions and proclaim innocence or push the guilt aside, and bury it deep somewhere. We will try to do any and everything we can to get rid of guilt. This is something that we get very good at... at a very young age, especially if we see our parents or other influential adults doing it.

Suppression of guilt feelings may lead to deep-seeded anger or abuse of alcohol or drugs or some other coverup. But the spirit of a man knows when it is not clean before the Lord. When the spirit of a man is not free from sin, guilt is present. Guilt feelings can create defensive attitudes leading to dysfunctional thinking and behaviors. These are important reasons to be free from guilt.

People that don't know the Lord (personally) have this feeling that God "might" be mad at them. Inwardly, their spirit knows they are not right or in right standing with God. They carry that feeling around. What they don't know is God wants to free them from that guilt and pain. The following two verses reveal that in the most powerful way!

For God did not send his Son into the world to condemn the world, but to save the world through him. **John 3:17**

God is not out to get us, but to save us, to free us! He isn't out to get us or bring condemnation which means "found guilty." He wants to wash our sins away!

But God demonstrates his own love for us in this: While we were yet sinners, Christ died for us. Since we have now been justified by the sacrifice of His death and blood, how much more shall we be saved from God's wrath through Jesus Christ! **Romans 5:8-9**

God has proven His love for us while we were still in a sinful state. That's how great His love is for us!

God does not point fingers. He says we have been justified and has given us a "not guilty" verdict. This is His gift to us. Although it is a free gift, He had to pay the price – with his life, through death on the cross. He took our punishment upon Himself. His sacrifice removes our sin and guilt and make us blameless.

God didn't send Jesus to get rid of guilt so that we could put each other back under it. He wants us free from guilt. This starts with receiving Jesus which frees us from sin. We need to break ourselves free from the chains of condemnation and guilt. These are a trap of the enemy to make us feel unworthy. Satan is a liar and a deceiver, and we need to recognize Satan for what he is.

Fasting awakens your spirit man to the areas in your life that He is not pleased with, areas where HE is not first, areas that we need to work on. It is a painful process indeed as we die to the flesh. As God reveals these things, we simply need to repent and move on. The sorrow may last for the night, but the joy comes in the morning. The freedom we can have when we are free of these burdens is indeed worth it. After we are delivered from these things we can then see the bondage we were in and truly rejoice!

Focus... On Him!

Our focus is to be on God at all times. Of course, that seems simple enough. But, the world (where Satan rules), quite bluntly stated, is out to get you and to keep you from anything that has to do with God. Many Christians unknowingly get caught up in the ways of the world. God even warns us of those who are *my people* who are doing the deceiving and distracting.

For among my people are found wicked men: they lay wait, as he that setteth snares; they set a trap, they catch men. **Jeremiah 5:26**

They shall not dwell in thy land, lest they make thee sin against me: for if thou serve their gods, it will surely be a snare unto thee. **Exodus 23:33**
And they served their idols: which were a snare unto them. **Psalm 106:36**

But they that will be rich fall into temptation and a snare, and into many foolish and hurtful lusts, which drown men in destruction and perdition. **1 Timothy 6:9**

Oh, The Distractions...

A distraction is anything that takes your mind off of what it is supposed to be on, anything that makes you feel discouraged so that you lose your peace and joy. Paul tells us in Philippians that if we have "lost" our peace, then our focus is off. This makes perfect sense because if we are focusing on what God wants us to be focusing on, the peace of God shall be with us.

Finally, brethren, whatsoever things are true, whatsoever things are honest, whatsoever things are just, whatsoever things are pure, whatsoever things are lovely, whatsoever things are of good report; if there be any virtue, and if there be any praise, think on these things. Those things, which ye have both learned, and received, and heard, and seen in me, do: and the God of peace shall be with you. **Philippians 4:8-9**

It does not matter if you are married or single, own a business, run a business, work at a business, have a family, ministry, classroom, farm, or whatever, there WILL be distractions in attempts to weaken, discourage, test and distract you from your focus. These distractions will probably come in all areas of your life. They will especially occur in what I call, "your weak areas." (Why would Satan attack your strengths? Satan never "plays" fair because it is not a game to him. He wants your soul and he wants it bad!)

As long as we are on earth, we will need the Lord's strength to stay on course and keep our focus on Him. The world, the flesh, and Satan want to prevent us from progressing down the Lord's perfect path.

We need to be more like David who wrote, *It is God who arms me with strength, and makes my way perfect,* **Psalm 18:32**. At times, when walking along our designated path of life, we get caught up in our circumstances like a trap laid by the enemy. When David experienced these traps, he cried out to God for strength he needed. *Pull me out of the net which they have secretly laid for me, For You are my strength,* **Psalm 31:4**. At other times along our path, the problem is not just a trap, but an all-out battle. Once again, David found the strength he needed in His Lord. *For You have armed me with strength for the battle; You have subdued under me those who rose up against me,* **Psalm 18:39.**

Your Focus is WHAT You Are Thinking About.

Often, the need for strength pertains to what is going on around us or within our own minds. The thoughts we are thinking, and the words we are expressing might (again) need to be realigned in the will of the Lord. David also knew how to turn to God for this essential strength as well. *Let the words of my mouth and the meditation of my heart be acceptable in Your sight, O LORD, my strength and my redeemer* (**Psalm 19:14**). When he weakened and stumbled in failure, David still knew where to turn for the only help that will ever prove sufficient. *My flesh and my heart fail; But God is the strength of my heart and my portion forever* (**Psalm 73:26**). Whenever you need strength, pray like David, *The LORD is my strength, in whom I will trust.*

*Casting down imaginations, and every high thing that exalteth itself against the knowledge of God, and bringing into captivity **every thought** to the obedience of Christ;* **2 Corinthians 10:5**

Watch and pray, that ye enter not into temptation: the spirit indeed is willing, but the flesh is weak. **Matthew 26:41**

Hungry

At one point during my research for this book, I thought the title of the book was going to be "Hungry." I believed that the book was to be about the importance of stirring our spiritual hunger for God, for our longing for Him and the Holy Spirit to fill the emptiness that resides in all of us.

This still is a very important concept of the book. We seem to have gotten so far off the tract in regards to what is really important to us. If God is our focus, none of these things (of the world and of the flesh) should matter.

As the hart panteth after the water brooks, so panteth my soul after thee, O God. My soul thirsteth for God, for the living God: when shall I come and appear before God? My tears have been my meat day and night, while they continually say unto me, Where is thy God? **Psalm 42:1-3**

Our faith begins with holy desires towards God and to communion with Him. Having a true and holy love to and for God is the power and motivation for our strive for godliness, the very life and soul of our faith. Without this love, all we do and say in His name are but an external performance – an empty shell.

Holy love thirsting in holy desires towards the Lord: "My soul panteth, thirsteth, for God, for nothing more than God, but still for more and more of Him."

When David wrote this Psalm, it was when he was debarred from his outward opportunities of waiting on

God, when he was banished to the land of Jordan, a great way off from the courts of God's house. Sometimes God has to teach us to know the worth of His mercies by removing us from them. By doing this, He stirs our appetite. We are apt to loathe manna when we have plenty of it, which will be very precious to us if ever we come to know the scarcity of it. When David was deprived of the inward comfort he used to have in God, he then longed for it. He mourned and went on panting.

Note that David writes his soul thirsts for the *living God*, not only in opposition to dead idols, the works of men's hands, but to all the dying comforts of this world, which perish in the using. Living souls can never take up their rest anywhere short of a living God. He longs to appear before God, to make himself known to him, as being conscious to himself of his own sincerity, to attend on him, as a servant appears before his master. Matthew Henry writes, *"To appear before God is as much the desire of the upright and sincere as it is the dread of the hypocrite."*

Also note that David writes that it is his *soul* that pants, his *soul* that thirsts. This shows us not only the sincerity, but the depth of his desire. He compares it to the panting of a hart (a deer) like a hunted buck, after the water-brooks. Thus earnestly does a gracious soul desire communion with God, thus impatient is it in the want of that communion, so impossible does it find it to be satisfied with anything short of that communion, and so insatiable is it in taking the pleasures of that communion when the opportunity of it returns, still thirsting after the full enjoyment of him in the heavenly kingdom.

In the last day, that great day of the feast, Jesus stood and cried, saying, If any man thirst, let him come unto me, and drink. He that believeth on me, as the scripture hath said, out of his belly shall flow rivers of living water. **John 7:37-38**

If you have ever had a time in your life which was extremely spiritually fulfilling, followed by a "dry spell," then you know what David is describing. If you have a devoted spiritual life of communion with God and Christ Jesus, and yet found there were times for whatever reason that you got off track, perhaps even due to the extended visitation of friends or family, or personal travel, etc., that you just felt like that daily communication wasn't there, you also know what David is talking about. There have been times where I just "miss" my Lord, I long for Him, even though He is right here all the time. He never leaves us, we leave His presence.

If you have never had a deep personal relationship with the Father and with Jesus, you may feel a sense that "there is something missing in my life." As our name is written in the Lamb's Book of Life, then that yearning is automatically instilled deep within us. It is the call of God. We are one of His. More than anything, He wants us to come home to Him and commune intimately with Him.

If we don't feel that deep hunger and yearning in our bones, then something is wrong; God is calling us to Him. While He has called us to holiness (Ephesians

1), if we are living in the flesh we may be numbed to the Holy Spirit, and that deep yearning cannot be satisfied, and God is the only one who can satisfy it.

If we eat snacks (often lacking nutritional value) all day long, we do not experience hunger when it comes to meal time, because we feel full. In a spiritual sense, we may think we are full (because we have been snacking on this or that unfulfilling whatever), and God will sometimes have to create a drought (perhaps trying circumstances) so we will hunger for Him. These are usually not the most pleasant times, but God has an important point to what He is bringing us through.

Paul, in Romans (8:7-8) talks about how the things of the flesh (self) cannot satisfy our spiritual needs (or be pleasing to God). These things provide only fleeting (if that, even) pleasure, or you can deceive yourself to believe that you are happy and at peace with your life, while the soul and spirit are dying, crying out to God.

You can deny it (your spiritual call), you can turn your back from it (knowingly, in outright rebellion or unknowingly, like a lost sheep), but God is there, always calling you. There is nothing in the world that can satisfy the things of God; No amount of money or wealth, no material thing, no amount of sex, no food, no relationship (no matter how perfect), no drug or amount of alcohol, or anything else that Satan will try to deceive us into thinking can satisfy our deep desire for God. No, nothing.

For those who live according to the flesh and are controlled by its unholy desires set their minds on and pursue those things which gratify the flesh, but those who are in the Spirit and are controlled by the desires of

61

*the Spirit set their minds on and seek those things which
gratify the Spirit.* **Romans 8:5** AMP

God will search out every lost sheep until he is
found. God will continue to call your name and wait
with more patience than any one of us can ever imagine. He waited for me, He will wait for you!

*O God, thou art my God; early will I seek thee: my
soul thirsteth for thee, my flesh longeth for thee in a dry
and thirsty land, where no water is.* **Psalm 63:1** (A Psalm
of David, when he was in the wilderness of Judah.)

*Ho, every one that thirsteth, come ye to the waters,
and he that hath no money; come ye, buy, and eat; yea,
come, buy wine and milk without money and without
price. Wherefore do ye spend money for that which is not
bread? and your labor for that which satisfieth not? hearken diligently unto me, and **eat ye that which is good,**
and let your soul delight itself in fatness. Incline your ear,
and come unto me: hear, and your soul shall live; and I
will make an everlasting covenant with you, even the sure
mercies of David.* **Isaiah 55:1-3**

What *Are* You Hungry For?

What we see most of the time (regardless of what
people SAY that the answer is) are of the world. All the
things that we desire, do or focus on to fill the emptiness cannot fill the "God-shaped hole" He put in all of
us. The things we try to fill it with include food, relationships with a lover, multiple lovers, spouse, spouses, family, personal gain or social status, money, work,
sex, alcohol, hobbies (such as gardening, music, cars,
collecting things), shopping (buying things - "He who

has the most toys wins"), etc.

When we see those who go from one relationship to the next, to the next, or one spouse to the next to the next, or one house to the next bigger house, to the next even bigger house with a pool, to the next with this and that and more, it is obvious (to us) that something is wrong. They seem to never be satisfied with anything. The things of the world simply cannot satisfy us. While as Christians, we know this, it is easy for us to get caught up in it all the same.

Some people thrive on busy-ness. Being busy, going here and there, errands, shopping, events, concerts, games, shows, parties, meetings, work, etc., never really accomplishing anything of true significance.

The years I lived in Southern California opened my eyes up to a lifestyle that one who had lived in North Dakota their entire life could not even imagine. Every evil of the world seemed so blatantly exaggerated and prevalent. There seemed to be more of what was deceit than there was truth. These things had become so commonplace, that to everyone around, these things seemed perfectly acceptable and even normal.

One thing that comes to mind is the huge expanse of the cosmetic surgery industry. This is essentially allowing "man" to surgically alter what God gave to you. I am referring to alterations not because of an accident (which we can be thankful that God gave the physicians the skill to do what they do), but simply because you want something better. It is very much a world which promotes vanity and the importance of outside appearances. There were times in the gym where I worked out that I was the only female in the entire place who did not have breast implants.

The surgical procedures available today to alter one's physical appearance is astounding. Both men and women have the choice of a new nose, chin, ears, or just about any other redesigned facial feature, calf implants, hair implants, liposuction, tummy tucks, chin tucks, butt tucks, and on and on. Breast implants were often not just installed once, but three, four and five times, creating larger and larger breasts each time. This reminds me of the story in Ezekiel about the two adulterous sisters who were infatuated with the exaggerated sexuality of the men. *For she doted upon their paramours, whose flesh is as the flesh of asses, and whose issue is like the issue of horses.* **Ezekiel 23:20**

It is like God is trying to show us how far off the (right) path we have gotten, to the point where it is even vulgar to Him, yet we still don't "get it."

There are certainly cities (such as Las Vegas and New Orleans) with a reputation for their sexual sin and lewdness, but what is "expected" in those cities can be found in every major city, as well as the sins of vanity and selfishness.

In metropolitan retail areas one can find nail salons on every street corner (next to the coffee houses), an abundance of spas and gyms to promote fitness, weight loss and detox. Today, many gyms are considered hot "pick-up" spots. Bars and nightclubs used to be the place where you would get "hit on" or find a date, now it's the gym and your local coffee house. Many people go to gyms there not to work out, but to socialize. I used to laugh at the girls spending more time on their hair and makeup in the bathroom than they did actually exercising. (Of course, they didn't want to work out too much or they would spoil their hair and make up!)

Day spas are popping up all over as a place to run away from "life" and be pampered for the day with a facial, massage, manicure, pedicure, body wrap, waxing, mineral-salted whirlpool and on and on. There are even special spas designed as a place to recover from cosmetic surgery so you can hide for a week or two so no one will (supposedly) know you had the surgery.

Gossip, course jokes, promiscuity, promiscuous dressing, sex outside of marriage, lawsuits, living off of credit cards, scams, alcohol and drug addictions (prescription and illegal), eating disorders, reliance upon therapists, fortune tellers, psychics and palm readers, and every other sort of "Sodom and Gamorrah" situation imaginable, have become so common that it all seems normal and acceptable to most people. Appearance is of the utmost importance; what car you drive, what kind of clothes and jewelry you wear, where you live, who your friends are, where you eat and socialize, etc. All of the external, superficial things in one's life are very, very important to people.

I lived in Southern California for about 8 years where this lifestyle is highly prevalent. I used to call it, "The land of the beautiful people." But none, or very little, was natural beauty, just fake (man-altered) beauty. Even the landscaping is meticulous, but it was "unnatural" as well, as most of that area is naturally dry desert and therefore, requires built-in irrigation systems to water all the transplanted foliage.

It was very difficult to find people of integrity, moral standard and modesty. If you lived near the beach, you had a constant flow of people 8 or 9 months of the year, rollerblading, skateboarding or biking past your house with little-to-nothing on. Intoxicated people, people who had no other desire in life than to have a good time, were always close by, encouraging all those around to join in on the fun. The social-scene, the party lifestyle, the bar-hopping, etc., was so prevalent, I often wondered if anyone worked or had a family. The topics of conversation revolved around where they went the night before and who else was there, what they were wearing, and who went home with whom. (It is amazing what you can learn when you go to a large salon to get your hair or nails done; most of the time I wanted to cover my ears!)

This is just an example of the degradation taking place just about everywhere, especially in the metropolitan areas. But, as you all probably know, it is far more exaggerated in some areas than others.

As I look back, I wonder why God had me there for those years. Maybe it was just to show me how messed up the world really is. I remember questioning some "Christians" who had lived in California quite a while, about what they thought about all "this" (sin, really is what is boils down to). Their response was, "Oh, you get used to it."

This is exactly the attitude that God is warning us about. This is apathy! We are NOT supposed to get used to it. We are to FLEE from it. We are NOT to associate in any way with it, lest we become contaminated ourselves. What do we do? It is true, sin is everywhere! It is on TV, billboards, magazines, radio, in the music, movies, malls, stores, internet, in our schools, libraries, and even in our churches.

One cannot claim to be a Christian and fully expect to go to heaven when the (continual) sin in one's life exists. You may say, "well, those people probably were not Christians." Well, I don't imagine that too many were. But, I believed that I was and yet was getting sucked into the ways of the world, even if I did not realize it at the time.

If you don't stand for something, you'll fall for everything.

No man can serve two masters: for either he will hate the one, and love the other; or else he will hold to the one, and despise the other. Ye cannot serve God and mammon. **Matthew 6:24**

Taste and See that the Lord is Good!

You may be thinking, we have to live here in the world, we have no choice. We have to work and be exposed to all sorts of things on a daily basis. This whole "death to self" thing, is so hard to do. This is what Paul wrote to the Corinthians.

Always bearing about in the body the dying of the Lord Jesus, that the life also of Jesus might be made manifest in our body. For we which live are always delivered unto death for Jesus' sake, that the life also of Jesus might be made manifest in our mortal flesh. So then death worketh in us, but life in you. We having the same spirit of faith, according as it is written, I believed,

67

*and therefore have I spoken; we also believe, and there-
fore speak; Knowing that he which raised up the Lord
Jesus shall raise up us also by Jesus, and shall present
us with you. For all things are for your sakes, that the
abundant grace might cause thanksgiving to overflow to
the glory of God.* **2 Corinthians 4:10-15**

Thank goodness for God's grace! *For which cause
we faint not; but though our outward man perish, yet the
inward man is renewed day by day. For our light affliction, which is but for a moment, worketh for us a far
more exceeding and eternal weight of glory; While we
look not at the things which are seen, but at the things
which are not seen: for the things which are seen are
temporal; but the things which are not seen are eternal.*
2 Corinthians 4:16-18

The Word of God...The Bread of Life!

Jesus was led by the Spirit into the wilderness for
40 days and scripture tells us that Satan tempted
Jesus for all 40 days. Satan even tried to kill Jesus as
he tried to convince him to jump from the the pinna-
cle of the temple (Luke 4:9). Satan will indeed do whatever he can to distract us and steal the time that is
meant for God. The scriptures tell us Jesus was hungry. Of course, He was, He was human.

While the degree of hunger varies greatly from one
individual to the next while fasting, the feeling of
hunger is inevitable at some point. When one goes
without eating, one also loses physical strength.
Fasting is a time of great weakness in many areas.
Going without food can create weakness, irritability,

depression, feelings of isolation, fear, anger and other human reactions that may seem to come out of nowhere (revealing just how human we are). As Peter denied Christ three times, we do not know how we may react when our hour of trial comes. (Luke 24:61) Prayer, for this reason, is very important at this time.

And said unto them, Why sleep ye? rise and pray, lest ye enter into temptation. **Luke 22:46**

Fasting is also to be a time of repentance and of cleansing. But as God reveals things He wants you to repent of, Satan will be right there to condemn you and shame you. While fasting we are likely to have feelings of unworthiness and question all sorts of things. You may wonder why is it so hard to go without food (mentally and physically) or even question your walk with God, your (impure) motives, times of backsliding, etc. God may remind you of "in the belly of the whale" times that you had stuffed away somewhere in shame. It is a time of nakedness as God strips you of all the things He wants you to get rid of.

This is why it is so important to spend as much time as possible in prayer and in studying and meditating on the Word at this time. *And the devil said unto him, If thou be the Son of God, command this stone that it be made bread. And Jesus answered him, saying, It is written, That man shall not live by bread alone, but by every word of God.* **Luke 4:3**

Bread does not just represent "food," it represents every reliance upon man, the world, and of self and the flesh. To God, our reliance upon these things is idolatry.

A fast (of any kind or length) that does not take you

out of your "normal life" and get you into the Word (more than your normal daily devotional, etc.), may not be worth doing in God's eyes. Fasting is a commitment to God to not simply give up food for a time, but to set your mind on Him and to get to know Him. How else do we get to know God, but by reading His Word and spending time with him?

Deuteronomy 8:3 says, *And he humbled thee...* (God had to humble them... show them that He was God and in control... and they were not.)

...and suffered thee to hunger, (Because of their disobedience, God needed to chastise them... as a father disciplines his son.)

God had a purpose for what He was doing, just as He has a purpose for us. He was trying to bless them, but in order to receive this blessing, God requires obedience to His Word. God wants to take care of us, to provide us with of all of our needs, but we must let Him (and quit doing things on our own).

As God took the Israelites through the wilderness to humble them, to discipline them, in order that He could bless them in freedom from their bondage from Pharaoh, so must we go through the same, as Christ Jesus has freed us from the bondages from our own sin. Satan is our bondsman and he will do whatever he can to keep us from (living in) our freedom. It is important that we search our lives and hearts for the things that God wants us to be freed of.

The Israelites had to let go of their idols, and we need to let go of ours. We need to let go of the past and let God heal us and redeem us so we can move into the great blessings that God has planned for us! Being a

Christian is about being FREE from the holds that Satan (our bondsman) not only had on us, but those he would try to put on us in the future. **We are FREE through Christ's death** as He has paid our debt in full. His death means life and FREEDOM for us!

But because the LORD loved you, and because he would keep the oath which he had sworn unto your fathers, hath the LORD brought you out with a mighty hand, and redeemed you out of the house of bondmen, from the hand of Pharaoh king of Egypt. **Deuteronomy 7:8**

Fasting and Focus

The following story in Zechariah is a very important lesson as to **how** God wants us to fast, to pray and even how we are to eat! In fasting and all prayer we **must** set ourselves as before the Lord, must see His eye upon us and have our focus on **Him.** In all we do, it should glorify the Father (not ourselves.)

This is a story told by the prophet Zechariah and the children of the captivity concerning fasting. They question God whether they should continue their solemn fasts which they had religiously observed during the 70 years of their captivity. The answer to this question was given not all at once, and actually several times, to signify its importance and seriousness. The prophet sharply corrects the people for the mismanagement of their fasts. He tells them to reform their lives, which would be the best way of fasting, and to take heed of those sins which brought those judgments upon them.

God told them their fasting was not done with a pure heart. *Speak unto all the people of the land, and to the priests, saying, When ye fasted and mourned in the fifth and seventh month, even those seventy years,* **did ye at all fast unto me, even to me?** *And when ye did eat, and when ye did drink,* **did not ye eat for yourselves, and drink for yourselves? Zechariah 7:5-6**

But they refused to hearken, *and pulled away the shoulder, and stopped their ears, that they should not hear. Yea,* **they made their hearts as an adamant stone,** *lest they should hear the law, and the words which the LORD of hosts hath sent in his spirit by the former prophets: therefore came a great wrath from the LORD of hosts. Therefore it is come to pass, that as he cried, and they would not hear; so they cried, and* **I would not hear, saith the LORD of hosts. Zechariah 7:10-13**

When we offer up our requests in prayer and fasting to God, it must be with a readiness to receive instructions from Him. AND, if we turn away from hearing His instruction, we cannot expect that our prayers and fasting will be acceptable to Him. We must pray, not only, "Lord, help me!" but, **"What do you want me to do for you?"**

Their fasting was not done correctly as they were not willing to be told of their faults, let alone to correct them. They were not focused on God in their fasting: *Did you at all fast unto me, even to me?* God knows all things. He is really saying, "You know very well that you did not at all fast to me," They may have appeared outwardly to be conducting their duty of fasting, but they were essentially only going through the motions as they were not including the life, and soul, and power of it.

*For thou shalt worship no other god:
for the LORD, whose name is Jealous,
is a jealous God.* Exodus 34:14

Was it to me, even to me? The repetition reveals the great deal of emphasis that God gives this issue. Fasting must be done for God, focusing upon Him, sincerely searching the scriptures as our rule, and His will for His glory.

To God, the way that they had been fasting was an insult. To fast, but not fast to God (with a sincere heart), was to mock and provoke Him, and could not be pleasing to Him.

Those that make fasting a coverup for sin, as Jezebel's fast, or to men for appearance sake like the Pharisees, or that only demonstrate outward expressions of humiliation while their hearts are unhumbled, as Ahab, are not fasting to God... and He knows it.

Further, it appears that they were as focused on themselves in their fasting as they were in their eating and drinking (v. 6): *When you did eat, and when you did drink, on other days did you not eat for yourselves and drink for yourselves?* Have you not always done as you please (serving yourself)? He is saying, "In your religious feasts and thanksgivings you were no more focused on God than you were in your fasts."

It also refers to their common meals; that they were not honoring God in their eating and drinking either; but that the service of their own needs was the center of all their actions.

God is saying that even what we eat and drink it

should not be to ourselves, but to the glory of God, that our bodies may be fit to serve our souls in His service.

So, whether you eat or drink, or whatever you do, do all to the glory of God. **1 Corinthians 10:31**

The principal thing they should have done in their fasting was left undone. They (and we also) should have searched the scriptures of the prophets, to see what was the ground of God's controversy with their fathers, and might have taken warning by their miseries not to continue in their sin. They asked, "Shall we continue to fast?" God tells them, "No, you must do that which you have not yet done; you must **repent of your sins** and **reform your lives.**"

The concept of our pursuit of holiness and the food choices we make and how we treat our bodies from a dietary or nutritional standpoint is foreign to most Christians today. The scripture in 1 Corinthians 10:31 is clear to me that we need to be treating our bodies as a temple of the Holy Spirit at all times, even in our food and beverage choices, as this will bring glory to God. So many of our food choices tear down the body leading to sickness and disease which does not glorify God. Eating like a pagan does not glorify God.

Our eating habits and our participation in fasting and a fasted life-style play a huge role in being obedient to God's instructions. *Be ye holy, for I am holy.*

It is God's desire that every part of us reflect Christ's true character to others, to our brothers and sisters in Christ and also to those who do not know Him. This is how we can serve Him.

Holiness

The Holiness of God

"Holy" means "set apart." God is set apart from us, from anyone who lives now, ever has or ever will. He is, in character, in perfection, in purity, in ability, in knowledge, set apart from everyone and everything. There are adjectives that pertain only to Him: Omniscient, Omnipotent, Omnipresent.

What is wisdom or knowledge without holiness, but craft and cunning? What is power without holiness, but tyranny, oppression, and cruelty?

God is *glorious in holiness* (Exodus 15:11) and this gives a luster, glory and perfection to all He does. Therefore, nothing of God can be exercised in a wrong manner, or to any bad purpose. His character and essence is infinite and unbounded. It cannot be greater than it is, and can neither be increased nor diminished.

God is morally perfect. *Let no one say when he is tempted, "I am tempted by God"; for God cannot be tempted by evil, nor does He Himself tempt anyone.* **James 1:13**

We are sinful and unholy and we live in an unclean, unholy society. How can we possibly understand and fully comprehend the holiness of God? How can we understand the power of God? The perfection? The awesomeness? We simply cannot. If we could we would not be living the lives most of us are. We would be so fearful and in such awe of his majesticness that

75

we would be devastated just as Isaiah was.

We cannot fully understand the holiness of God, so we compromise. We have compromised our God to the point that we have corrupted our whole religion.

We want a God who loves us unconditionally, who will make us comfortable (bless us and provide for all our needs), who is a "feel good" God, but we don't want to hear about how God is calling us to perfection, to holiness, and about the power and wrath of God. We say, "that's old fashioned," if told dancing, gambling, movies and our ways of dressing and talking are immoral. We say, "God accepts us as we are" when told we need to stop doing this or that. We need to wake up and realize that we cannot even claim to be a Christian and fully expect to enter the Holy gates of heaven while continuing a life of sin and disobedience.

✦ How can we continually feed the body junk food (that does not nourish the body but weaken it) and claim it is respecting the Holy Temple of God?

✦ How is continually stuffing yourself (gluttony) to the point of discomfort pleasing to the Father?

✦ How is mistreating your children (as well as not disciplining them properly when they misbehave) raising a "Christian" family? Or having an apathetic attitude thinking that "my kids are better than most."

✦ How is using the Lord's name in vain (even worse yet, in front of your children and on the way home from church, no less) honoring God?

◆ How is a wife submitting to her husband if she is doing things that affect the whole family with out even asking him, in service to God?

◆ How is staying home to watch TV, when the church was asking for someone to bring baked goods to raise money for the poor or for volunteers to visit the sick or to help grow and serve God's family?

◆ How is gossip pleasing to God's ears? How does accusing your brothers and sisters in Christ behind their backs edify the body of Christ?

Do you think that God does not see these things? Do you think that this behavior will be acceptable in heaven? Absolutely not! We need to be preparing ourselves NOW, before we get there. How else will God know if we are 100% for Him?

Feed the flock of God which is among you, taking the oversight thereof, not by constraint, but willingly; not for filthy lucre, but of a ready mind; **1 Peter 5:2**

Let us be glad and rejoice, and give honor to him: for the marriage of the Lamb is come, and his wife hath made herself ready. **Revelation 19:7**

And I John saw the holy city, new Jerusalem, coming down from God out of heaven, prepared as a bride adorned for her husband. **Revelation 21:2**

God is the ONLY one that matters. He knows our heart. He knows if we are a person of integrity who he can say to, *well done, good and faithful servant* **(Matthew 5: 21)** or if he will say:

Depart from me, ye cursed, into everlasting fire, pre-
pared for the devil and his angels: For I hungered, and
ye gave me no meat: I was thirsty, and ye gave me no
drink: I was a stranger, and ye took me not in: naked,
and ye clothed me not: sick, and in prison, and ye visit-
ed me not. Then shall they also answer him, saying,
Lord, when saw we thee an hungered, or athirst, or a
stranger, or naked, or sick, or in prison, and did not min-
ister unto thee? Then shall he answer them, saying,
Verily I say unto you, Inasmuch as ye did it not to one of
the least of these, ye did it not to me. And these shall go
away into everlasting punishment: but the righteous into
life eternal. **Matthew 25:41-45**

We see too many pastors afraid to preach about what God is really calling them to preach about because it might stir up the people, it might make them uncomfortable, it might step on some toes (and it might affect next week's offering).

We can read about His holiness in the scriptures, but we can't hardly identify with what it is like to be sinless. We cannot comprehend God's holiness and this is the reason we are so defiant, so disobedient, so selfish, so idolatrous, so selfish, so critical of others. When we begin to understand the true God (through the process of sanctification), we will start seeing the truth about our sinfulness and how horrible the sin in our life is. We will then begin to see how we have broken God's heart and how we have grieved the Holy Spirit.

We have so corrupted our own religion that we do not even understand the principles of worship and what worship is.

But in vain they do worship me, teaching for doctrines the commandments of men. **Matthew 15:9**

Too many people go to church and sing along, not really paying attention to the words that are coming out. Many people are looking around to see who else is there... and who is not. This is supposed to be an intimate time between you and the Father. We should have our eyes closed and our heart focused on nothing else but Him. We should be asking for forgiveness for our sinfulness and our unworthiness to come before Him. David wrote we are to *Enter into his gates with thanksgiving, and into his courts with praise: be thankful unto him,* and bless his name. **Psalm 100:4**

Do we really comprehend the sovereignty of God? This is his absolute right to do all things according to his own good pleasure **(Daniel 4:25, 35; Romans 9:15-23; 1 Timothy 6:15; Revelation 4:11).**

The absence of our understanding of the holiness of God is rebellion, is irreverent, is our own pride, and is even idolatry. *Thou shalt have no other gods before me.* **Exodus 20:3**

When we pray and when we worship, we need to first acknowledge the holiness of God. Jesus taught us to pray: *Therefore pray ye: Our Father which art in heaven, Hallowed be thy name.* **Matthew 6:9**

He is so Holy that in our sinful state, we cannot enter into God's presence. Isaiah said, *"Woe is me! I am lost, for I am a man of unclean lips, and I live among a people of unclean lips; yet my eyes have seen the King, the LORD of hosts!" Then one of the seraphims flew to*

79

me, holding a live coal that had been taken from the altar with a pair of tongs. The seraphims touched my mouth with it and said: "Now that this has touched your lips, your guilt has departed and your sin is blotted out." **Isaiah 6:4-7**

When Moses asked God if he could see Him, God answered, ***Thou canst not see my face: for there shall no man see me and live.***

And the LORD said, Behold, there is a place by me, and thou shalt stand upon a rock: And it shall come to pass, while my glory passeth by, that I will put thee in a clift of the rock, and will cover thee with my hand while I pass by: And I will take away mine hand, and thou shalt see my back parts: but my face shall not be seen. **Exodus 33:20-23**

While I am so thankful that our new covanant through the blood of Jesus allows us to enter the throne room in rightousness, we seem to have lost our holy fear (reverence) of God. We often take forgranted the sacrificial price that was paid for us. So much irreverence is visible even inside the church; hats are seen on men, women are dressed in short tight skirts or other immodest manner, young undisciplined children are disruptive, or the teens not even required to sit with their family, talk and pass notes through the service. In the old testament, rebellious children were put to death.

We can never stand in the presence of God; we would be consumed with the horribleness of our own sin; we would be devastated just as the prophet Habakkuk was as he stood in the presence of God.

Habakkuk records that he trembled, his lips quivered and he came into the realization of how sinful he was.

When I heard (God speak), ***my belly trembled; my lips quivered at the voice: rottenness entered into my bones, and I trembled in myself.*** **Habakkuk 3:16**

We should have the same reverence, where we would tremble and be humbled at our own sinfulness in the presence of God. Only through Jesus can we approach our Holy God in confidence.

Therefore, since we have a great high priest who has gone through the heavens, Jesus the Son of God, let us hold firmly to the faith we profess. For we do not have a high priest who is unable to sympathize with our weaknesses, but we have one who has been tempted in every way, just as we are--yet was without sin. Let us then approach the throne of grace with confidence, so that we may receive mercy and find grace to help us in our time of need. **Hebrews 4:14-16** NIV

Even the holiness of Christ Jesus exposed the "unholiness" of the Pharisees. They felt so threatened by Him they had to kill Him.

Why have we become so irreverent, so complacent? It's like we accept the parts that we like about God (the love and forgiveness) and don't want to hear about His wrath, His power, His holiness. How did we get so prideful?

O ye sons of men, how long will ye turn my glory into shame? how long will ye love vanity, and seek after leasing? Selah. **Psalm 4:2**

Special Brownies! (Author Unknown)

Many parents are hard pressed to explain to their youth why some music, movies, books, and magazines are not acceptable material for them to bring into the home or to listen to or see.

One parent came up with an original idea that is hard to refute. The father listened to all the reasons his children gave for wanting to see a particular PG-13 movie. It had their favorite actors. Everyone else was seeing it. Even church members said it was great. It was only rated PG-13 because of the suggestion of sex. The language was pretty good--the Lord's name was only used in vain three times in the whole movie.

The teens did admit there was a scene where a building and a bunch of people were blown up, but the violence was just the normal stuff. It wasn't too bad. And, even if there were a few minor things, the special effects were fabulous and the plot was action packed.

However, even with all the justifications the teens made for the PG-13 rating, the father still wouldn't give in. He didn't even give his children a satisfactory explanation for saying, "No." He just said, "No!"

A little later on that evening the father asked his teens if they would like some brownies he had baked. He explained that he'd taken the family's favorite recipe and added a little something new. The children asked what it was.

The father calmly replied that he had added dog poop. However, he quickly assured them, it was only a little bit. All other ingredients were gourmet quality and he had taken great care to bake the brownies at the precise temperature for the exact time. He was sure the brownies would be superb.

Even with their father's promise that the brownies were of almost perfect quality, the teens would not take any. The father acted surprised. After all, it was only one small part that was causing them to be so stubborn. He was certain they would hardly notice it. Still the teens held firm and would not try the brownies.

The father then told his children how the movie they wanted to see was just like the brownies. Our minds trick us into believing that just a little bit of evil won't matter. But, the truth is even a little bit of poop makes the difference between a great treat and something disgusting and totally unacceptable.

The father went on to explain that even though the movie industry would have us believe that most of today's movies are acceptable fare for adults and youth, they are not.

Now, when this father's children want to see something that is of questionable material, the father merely asks them if they would like some of his special dog poop brownies. That closes the subject.

All things are lawful, but not all things are profitable. All things are lawful, but not all things edify.
1 Corinthians 10:23

Opposite of Holy: SIN

In order to separate those (The Israelites) who God chose as His children, He gave them "The Law" which contained strict rules about the manner of ways which God wanted the people to be "clean." Things that were deemed "unclean" were to be avoided until they were made clean.

Sinning against God makes us unclean! *Thus they were defiled by their own works, And played the harlot by their own deeds.* **Psalm 106:39**

But we are all like an unclean thing, And all our righteousness are like filthy rags; We all fade as a leaf, And our iniquities, like the wind, Have taken us away. **Isaiah 64:6**

The Old Testament serves as a teacher for us as we examine the concept of holiness in the New Covenant we have with the Christ. Sanctification in the New Testament means that you are set apart from sin, and dedicated to the service of Christ:

I beseech you therefore, brethren, by the mercies of God, that you present your bodies a living sacrifice, holy, acceptable to God, which is your reasonable service. And do not be conformed to this world, but be transformed by the renewing of your mind, that you may prove what is that good and acceptable and perfect will of God. **Romans 12:1-2**

Sanctification under the new covenant is of a higher order: *For if the blood of bulls and goats and the ashes of a heifer, sprinkling the unclean, sanctifies for the purifying of the flesh, how much more shall the blood of Christ, who through the eternal Spirit offered Himself without spot to God, cleanse your conscience from dead works to serve the living God? And for this reason He is the Mediator of the new covenant, by means of death, for the redemption of the transgressions under the first covenant, that those who are called may receive the promise of the eternal inheritance.* **Hebrews 9:13-15**

To be Holy is to be sinless, perfect, to be pleasing to God. Christ was the only true holy man to walk the earth. *But with the precious blood of Christ, as of a lamb without blemish and without spot:* **1 Peter 1:19**

Holiness denotes the manifestation of the quality of Christ in our personal conduct. Romans 1:4, of the absolute "holiness" of Christ in the days of His flesh, which distinguished Him from all merely human beings. *And declared to be the Son of God with power, according to the spirit of holiness, by the resurrection from the dead:* **Romans 1:4**

As believers we are to be *perfecting holiness in the fear of God* (**2 Corinthians 7:1**). We should all be growing toward perfection, to develop likeness to Christ. Holiness is a manifestation of true Christian character which involves grace, humility, truth, integrity, righteousness and a right relation to God. Holiness and godliness are similar in meaning, denoting a sacred character of reverence to God.

Complete holiness is the desire and duty of every

true Christian. Here are the two parts of this holiness:

1. We must be holy, and be so in all manner of conversation; in all civil and religious affairs, in every condition, towards all people, friends and enemies; in all interactions and business.

2. We must be holy, as God is holy: we must imitate him, though we can never equal him. He is perfectly, unchangeably, and eternally holy; and we should aspire after the same.

That he might present it to himself a glorious church, not having spot, or wrinkle, or any such thing; but that it should be holy and without blemish. **Ephesians 5:27**

As obedient children, not fashioning yourselves according to the former lusts in your ignorance: But as he which hath called you is holy, so be ye holy in all manner of conversation; Because it is written, Be ye holy; for I am holy. **1 Peter 1:16**

Paul's letter to the Ephesians tells us that we were elected and predestined to be holy. Election means that some were chosen out of all mankind – separated and distinguished. Predestination refers also to the purpose for what we are designed for; particularly the adoption of children, it being the purpose of God that in due time we should become His adopted children, and so have a right to all the privileges of the inheritance. Predestined also means this act of love occurred before the foundation of the world; not only before Adam and Eve, but before the world had a beginning.

We are not chosen that we *should* be holy; but

because He foresaw we *would* be holy, and because He determined to make us so. The sanctification, as well as salvation, is the result of the counsels of divine love. Holiness is not to be merely external and in outward appearance, so as to prevent blame from men, but internal and real. Because God knows our true heart, He will know. Holiness is to flow out of us as love to God and to our fellow man. Love is the principle of all true holiness.

According as he hath chosen us in him before the foundation of the world, that we should be holy and without blame before him in love. **Ephesians 1:4**

In the book of Haggai, the Lord was chastising His people about how they had let their hearts, their attitudes and their character be influenced by those that did not know or care about God or His ways. They had moved away from God and they had become contaminated. This is what the Apostle Paul is saying to the church of Corinth. *Do not be misled or deceived: Bad company corrupts good character.* The Amplified version reads, *Do not be so deceived and misled! Evil companionship (communion, associations) corrupt and deprave good morals and character.* **1 Corinthians 15:33**

Why did he say "do not be deceived?" Remember, those who are being deceived **do not know it.** We often hear people say things like, "Listening to this (secular) music isn't going to hurt me. Watching and listening to profanity, sex, and violence on TV and the movies isn't going to hurt me. Listening to crude jokes just goes in one ear and out the other." This is not true. These things make imprints on the heart and mind. They numb us. They harden the heart and deaden us to the Spirit. The truth is, they contaminate us. The world's influence will contaminate you. We are to live in the world, but not of the world.

The world is contaminated and we should want to influence people toward God and for good. We are called (Ephesians 1:4) to be holy, to be set apart from those in the world. To be different. *And be not conformed to this world: but be ye transformed by the renewing of your mind, that ye may prove what is that good, and acceptable, and perfect, will of God.* **Romans 12:2**

The things of the world numb us. They harden the heart and deaden us to the Spirit. The truth is, they contaminate us.

Most evils start by simply getting their foot into the crack of the door. Once it has the door open, it just keeps coming in. If it increases slowly enough, it may not be even noticed for a long while until it is too late and what started out as something which may seem insignificant at the time, gets a foothold, on its way to becoming a stronghold.

If you allow a sexually suggestive photo or calender into the house (or garage), over time this can turn into a library of pornographic magazines and videos. What starts out as a curious glance to a horoscope can explode into hundreds of dollars or more spent on psychics, palm readers, etc.

The same principle applies for what you allow in your place of work. Frequently allowing others to speak profane language around you could eventually cause it to start coming out of you. If it doesn't hurt your ears and bother your spirit, there is something wrong. When you are living in the flesh, the sensitivity to the Holy Spirit deadens your spirit.

Because the carnal mind is enmity against God: for it is not subject to the law of God, neither indeed can be. So then they that are in the flesh cannot please God. But ye are not in the flesh, but in the Spirit, if so be that the Spirit of God dwell in you. Now if any man have not the Spirit of Christ, he is none of his. And if Christ be in you, the body is dead because of sin; but the Spirit is life because of righteousness. But if the Spirit of him that raised up Jesus from the dead dwell in you, he that raised up Christ from the dead shall also quicken your mortal bodies by his Spirit that dwelleth in you. **Romans 8:7-11**

We (in our flesh) cannot satisfy our needs of the Spirit, while that is our eternal longing. We will search and search, going from one thing to another searching, but God is the only one who can fill the hunger.

We must be very careful to what we expose ourselves to. Many things will stir up the flesh just by proximity. In Haggai it talks about how important it is to keep thyself from what is evil.

Thus saith the LORD of hosts; Ask now the priests concerning the law, saying, If one bear holy flesh in the skirt of his garment, and with his skirt do touch bread, or pottage, or wine, or oil, or any meat, shall it be holy? And the priests answered and said, No. Then said Haggai, If one that is unclean by a dead body touch any of these, shall it be unclean? And the priests answered and said, It shall be unclean. Then answered Haggai, and said, So is this people, and so is this nation before me, saith the LORD; and so is every work of their hands; and that which they offer there is unclean. **Haggai 2:11-14**

Live as children of obedience to God; do not conform yourselves to the evil desires (that governed you) in your former ignorance (when you did not know the requirements of the Gospel.) **1 Peter 1:14** AMP

Teachers of young children can easily tell what kind of language is used at home by their parents and older siblings, because the same thing comes out of them. We become what we are exposed to.

We are surrounded by a multitude of these influences everywhere and it continually gets worse.

Instead of praying for and respecting those in positions of authority (as we are commanded) they are commonly ridiculed on the internet by comedians and the media. Sexual promiscuity and fornication is now common on television... and at any time of day (not just after nine at night). Many TV shows, magazines, movies, video games, internet sites, etc. promote promiscuity, adultery, fornication, homosexuality, fashion, glamour, physical appearance, materialism, violence, vulgar language, profanity, course joking, partial nudity and even nudity. Everyone justifies that it's no big deal - it's just entertainment. It is not! We should closely guard our ear gate, eye gate and flee from such things!

Horror movies, action movies and those which portray a lot of violence, are also something to be very cautious about. This also applies to video games which glorify violence and evil. Viewing these numbs and desensitizes us to their reality and the evil of their reality. Books, television shows and movies about witchcraft, cults, demon-possessed people or houses, etc. are not acceptable entertainment and cannot be assumed harmless. Demons can and do possess people, houses, trees, animals and can abide anywhere evil has been committed. To glorify these things of evil is contrary to what the Bible instructs. These are no more acceptable entertainment than are shows with crude language, adulterous affairs, murder, stealing, and etc.

I will set no wicked thing before mine eyes: I hate the work of them that turn aside; it shall not cleave to me. **Psalm 101:3**

I have found that I cannot watch many movies or television shows that I enjoyed even 4 or 5 years ago. I recall as a young teenager that I could not watch the movies (such as *Amityville Horror, Halloween*, etc.) that my friends enjoyed because they disturbed my spirit to such a great degree. At that time I thought there was something wrong with me, but now I realize that the purity level of a child is something we should all desire. Jesus said, *Verily I say unto you, Whosoever shall not receive the kingdom of God as a little child, he shall not enter therein.* **Mark 10:15**

As we get more involved in the world, we become desensitized to the things (evil) of the world. As we begin to pull back from the world, the more in tune we can get with the Holy Spirit and what He tells us is evil and what to flee from.

Do not be deceived. Just because many of these things are "common, popular or accepted" in the world does not mean they are no less damaging, and not the cause of greater destruction and death than anyone will ever know until God one day opens all mankind's eyes to this truth.

Holiness is an ongoing and progressive pursuit of inward change that the Holy Spirit will help us accomplish as we seek the Lord and His help. All blessings of God flow toward the heart that seeks Him and His ways. We experience joy over our fellowman because of our rightousness. **(Hebrews 1:9)**

The Bible clearly tells us to turn from evil: *Turn ye again now every one from his evil way, and from the evil of your doings, and dwell in the land that the LORD hath given unto you and to your fathers for ever and ever.* **Jeremiah 25:5**

Say unto them, As I live, saith the Lord GOD, I have no pleasure in the death of the wicked; but that the wicked turn from his way and live: turn ye, turn ye from your evil ways; for why will ye die, O house of Israel? **Ezekiel 33:11**

Abstain from all appearance of evil. **1 Timothy 5:22** Abstaining from all appearance of evil will help prevent us from being deceived with false doctrines.

Corruption in the heart, and evil practices allowed in our life will greatly tend to promote fatal errors in the mind. Purity of heart, and integrity of life, will dispose men to receive the truth and the love of it. We should therefore abstain from evil, and all appearances of evil, from sin, and that which looks like sin, leads to it, and borders upon it. He who is close to the appearances of sin, who does not turn his back on the occasions of sin, and who does not avoid the temptations and approaches to sin, will not long abstain from the actual commission of sin.

If a group of individuals (you may consider friends) you socialize with has questionable behavior; tend to gossip, complain, degrade their spouses, use improper language, allow inappropriate behavior by their children, etc., tell off-color jokes, overuse their credit cards, don't pay their bills on time, cheat on their income taxes, etc., but you feel that you don't do these things, you are wrong to think that they are not influencing you. If you associate with these people long enough, you are likely to start behaving the same way as they do.

A friend of mine has a son who is very gifted athletically. I keep encouraging him to train with someone who is better that he is. Otherwise, his training partner will not challenge him to improve, but instead may hold him back. I learned this in my many years of training in the gym. If you want to improve, you will want your training partner to pull you up to their level. It is the same in the world and the church. The people you hang out with will either challenge you to grow in God, hold you back, or pull you back into the world.

It has also been said that one cannot grow spiritually beyond the level of their pastor or mentor. IF they are not challenging you to grow spiritually, you may need to reconsider some things. More than once I have had to walk out of a church service because of inappropriate course "jokes" told from the pulpit. I knew the Holy Spirit was grieved and could not agree and allow that evil spirit operating there to influence me.

This is also why it is so important to monitor who your children are spending their time with. The behavior of your children's friends is likely to become the behavior of your child.

Discernment (in a maturation of our understanding) is something we (Christians) need in order to determine what is good and evil, true or false. *For every one that useth milk is unskillful in the word of righteousness: for he is a babe. But strong meat belongeth to them that are of full age, even those who by reason of use have their senses exercised to discern both good and evil.* **Hebrews 5:13-14**

Avoiding even the appearance of evil is also important. We're not to give others the opportunity to doubt the sincerity of our faith by our actions, even if we know the actions to be innocent. We do not want to lead others astray by what may appear to be wrong. You should not have to explain your actions; they should speak for themselves.

If we are to turn from it, we need to know what it is. So what is evil? Evil is sin. To sin is to wander from the law of God, to violate God's law. It is disobedience.

It is anything that is flesh or carnal, which denotes mere human nature apart from divine influence, and therefore prone to sin and opposed to God.

The flesh is considered the seat of sin in man.

For all that is in the world, the lust of the flesh, and the lust of the eyes, and the pride of life, is not of the Father, but is of the world. **1 John 2:16**

Watch and pray, that ye enter not into temptation: the spirit indeed is willing, but the flesh is weak. **Matthew 26:41**

Galatians 5 is pretty clear: *Now the works of the flesh are manifest, which are these; Adultery, fornication, uncleanness, lasciviousness, Idolatry, witchcraft, hatred, variance, emulations, wrath, strife, seditions, heresies, Envyings, murders, drunkenness, revellings, and such like: of the which I tell you before, as I have also told you in time past, that they which do such things shall not inherit the kingdom of God.* **Galatians 5:19-21**

You ask, but didn't Christ die for our sins? Of course He did. Our sins are forgiven, but He clearly instructs us to *sin no more.* (**John 5:14** and **John 8:11**) He is saying that you cannot "claim" to be a Christian and continue in these behaviors. He is saying you are either *For Him or against Him!*

And that repentance (to turn away from, a change of mind) *and remission* (forgiveness) *of sins should be preached in his name among all nations, beginning at Jerusalem.* **Luke 24:47**

Conviction and Grace

We all struggle and get caught up in the battle between the flesh and the spirit. The flesh (the corrupt and carnal part of us) lusts (struggles with strength) against the spirit opposing all the motions of the spirit, and resists everything that is spiritual. The spirit (the renewed part of us) strives against the flesh, and opposes the will and desire of it so we do not or cannot do the things that we would like to according to the flesh. The convictions of the Holy Spirit would suppress our corruptions; however, our corruptions (sins) silence our convictions. In all renewed (those with their old heart replaced with a new heart of Christ), there is a continual struggle between the old nature and the new nature. This struggle (as we win some and we lose some) is what teaches us the concept of the grace of God. This exercise will continue as long as we are in this world.

God Calls Us to Holiness... For Our Own Good

As we realize the holiness of God and His law is revealed to us in His Word, we start to realize how pathetic we are, how much we fall short. As we progress in our personal walk towards holiness, we will come to hate our own sin (**Psalm 119: 104**) as it is revealed to us and to delight in the law of God (**Romans 7:22**). We will realize that these laws are not a burden, but are for our own good, for our protection and for the good of all men.

Just as a child does not understand *why* he cannot play in the street or with matches, or with the buttons on the stove when told not to, we do not always understand WHY we are supposed to do as God commands. We do not understand how much pain it would cause a mother to have her son or husband killed; the guilt and loss you would feel if you had an abortion; how the soul is damaged and that ungodly soul ties are created when sexual intimacy occurs outside of marriage; how a child would feel to grow up without both parents if one abandons the family; how a child feels to grow up abused or neglected; how greed, covetousness, jealousy, manipulation and lies destroy friendships and families. Sin leads to more sin and more woundings.

What God commands of us is to protect our own selves and others from the deep woundings that sin causes. While sin separates us from God, the deep woundings within us caused by sin also separate us from God as these woundings create walls. Walls are built to protect ourselves from the pain and agony of those wounds, and of ever experiencing that pain again. Wall building is usually not a conscious effort, but a natural (human) reaction. We rarely know the walls are there. Subconsciously, we think, "as long as I don't let anyone in (through the walls), I can't get hurt again."

We do not like to suffer, we do not like the pain and agony of any emotional wounding of any kind. When we experience something traumatic, at any age, it is a natural reaction to want to prevent it from ever happening again. Some people do not even know how to deal with emotional issues because instead of dealing with and going through the pain, the issues are suppressed and walls are built to shut off the experience of any feeling what-so-ever.

If someone points out that the walls are there, denial, pride, stubbornness and fear, often keep the walls up. We can come up with all sorts of excuses to keep our walls up.

Common Wall Builders:

Unforgiveness

Grief (loss of loved one, etc.)

Childhood abuse, neglect, abandonment

Divorce

Divorce of parents

Tragedy (loss of house, business, etc.)

Serious personal injury or illness

Unmet needs (love, security)

Health problems

It is a common problem to bury the pain of these woundings instead of dealing with them and letting them heal. This reaction is one of fear and lack of trust in God.

God allows us to go through trials for a reason. (He does not put us through them.) *And we know that all things work together for good to them that love God, to them who are the called according to his purpose* (**Romans 8:28**). He is often trying to teach us something. (*A productive tree He prunes to produce even more.*) Sometime these trials may be a consequence of our own sin (as God is trying to teach us something).

There hath no temptation (trial or burden) taken you but such as is common to man: but God is faithful, who will not suffer you to be tempted above that ye are able; but will with the temptation also make a way to escape, that ye may be able to bear it. **1 Corinthians 10:13**

Instead of going through the pain and letting God heal us, we stuff it.

God tells us how to deal with all things (including the deep woundings of our soul); we need to turn to Him. We need to put and leave these things at His feet and let Him heal us. But, instead of going through the pain and healing, we "stuff it," meaning, we deny that we have been hurt, shut it out of our mind, not allowing our-selves to think about it, or pretend that it's no big deal and sweep it under the rug and move on. Consequently, years after "stuffing" everything, the result is an over-whelming state of unrest (lack of peace) and deep-seated feelings of depression, anger, unworthiness or disap-pointment (and most likely, health problems). Satan will use anything he can to beat you down and keep you from seeing the way to true peace. Many men are taught that "men don't cry" or "men don't show emotion" and many cultures encourage both men and women to "stuff" and hide emotional pain.

If there are issues in your past that still upset you when you think or talk about them, even if you feel that you have forgiven all individuals involved, you have not allowed God to heal you of the pain those incidents caused you. If it still "hurts" (causes you emotional pain to think about it), God's not done with you yet.

It is no wonder that such a high percentage of people are placed on anti-depressant medications. The problem of anti-depressant over-prescription is a huge problem today and the number of people taking them is staggering. Most of these (Prozac, Celexa, Sinequan, Paxil, Luvox, Zoloft, etc.) are SSRIs (selective serotonin reuptake inhibitors) and are highly addictive with numerous side effects. SSRIs increase the level of serotonin, a "feel good" hormone, in the brain.

Anti-depressants are enthusiastically accepted by the public looking for ways to deal with our stress-filled, anxiety-over-run "life." This reminds me of "feel good" anti-anxiety drugs of the 1960's and '70s, the benzodiazepines (Ativan, Valium, Xanax, etc.) that were widely promoted as safe and effective. It is now clear that benzodiazepine overuse and dependence was there all the time, though not revealed and/or obscured. Given the widespread assumption (until the mid-1980's) that benzodiazepines presented virtually no risk of dependence, doctors instead assumed that people took them for years because they really worked. Notice any similarities?

These comments were taken from Mayo Clinic Women's HealthSource: *SSRIs don't automatically make you "happy" or eliminate life's ups and downs. They don't replace the need for psychotherapy. But when taken with care and monitored by your doctor, SSRIs can help you deal more effectively with what life sends your way.*

This statement represents such a good example of how the world has such a simple solution (anti-Christ) for life's ups and downs. Why would anyone need God when you have Prozac?

The same principle applies to Ritalin (Methylphenidate), the prescription drug now commonly given to "active" children. With so many households with two parents working, or where there is only one parent in existence, and so many other (apparently more important) distractions from the proper raising and discipline of children today, no wonder so many parents are giving in to the world's solution of the day; drugs. Yep, drug the kids, that's the answer.

Methylphenidate is a central nervous system (CNS) stimulant. It has effects similar to, but more potent than, caffeine and less potent than amphetamines (such as cocaine). It has a notably calming effect on hyperactive children and a "focusing" effect on those with ADHD.

Ritalin™ is considered a Class II Drug and a controlled substance. Other drugs in this category are those such as cocaine, methamphetamine and methadone. A drug becomes a controlled substance when it has the potential for abuse and /or addiction. According to PAR (Parents Against Ritalin™) it is not uncommon in many classrooms today to find the percentage of children on Ritalin™ to be 25% or greater and the numbers are climbing.

There are many potentially damaging side-effects to Ritalin™, yet most parents don't know what else to do except to give their child the medication.

After we examine ourselves and remove the sin in our own life, we need to do the same with our entire family, our church family, our community and eventually the entire nation. Individuals of high moral and Christian conduct need to be positioned in places of leadership (teachers, pastors, elders, mayors, congressmen, etc.) (What a blessing it is to now have a Godly president in the White House!) These are the people that will be teaching and training our children. These individuals will have great influence upon us even if we do not realize its direct impact at all times.

Holiness and Diet

You may wonder what holiness has to do with diet and the things we eat. Remember, holiness is about our spirit, our diet (the food that we eat) is about flesh. Daniel served as a great example to show us how important it is to have a diet which is not focused upon what we might think tastes good (focusing on our fleshly desires), but a diet to promote good health.

But Daniel purposed in his heart that he would not defile himself with the portion of the king's meat, nor with the wine which he drank: therefore he requested of the prince of the eunuchs that he might not defile himself. **Daniel 1:8**

God blessed Daniel *with knowledge and skill in all learning and wisdom: and Daniel had understanding in all visions and dreams.* **Daniel 1:17**

When I was studying Daniel one day, God showed me how even though the diet that Daniel chose to eat (vegetables and water) is often referred to as "The Daniel Fast", that it was not really a "fast." This was the way that he chose to eat.

The prince of the eunuchs said unto Daniel, I fear my lord the king, who hath appointed your meat and your drink: for why should he see your faces worse lik-

ing than the children which are of your sort? then shall ye make me endanger my head to the king. Then said Daniel to Melzar, whom the prince of the eunuchs had set over Daniel, Hananiah, Mishael, and Azariah, Prove thy servants, I beseech thee, ten days; and let them give us pulse to eat, and water to drink. **Daniel 1:10-12**

So the fast was done simply to prove to Melzar that it was in their best interest of health.

After the 10 day trial, they appeared healthier and stronger than all the children which did eat the king's meat (Daniel 1:15). In addition, *in all matters of wisdom and understanding, that the king enquired of them, he found them ten times better than all the magicians and astrologers that were in all his realm.* **Daniel 1:20**

And then Daniel continued this diet... *even unto the first year of king Cyrus* (thought to be two years), **Daniel 1:21.**

Our diet today seems to be way off focus. I recently learned that candy is commonly given to children in Sunday School at many churches as treats, prizes and rewards. While I don't understand why children need to be given any motivation or reward for learning God's word, I am especially bothered with this misuse of something that does not even belong in the church or the human body. This practice contributes not only to unhealthy eating habits, health problems and obesity, but is a silent message that they should be rewarded for every time they do something for God.

Food and eating are necessary to sustain life. They are also pleasurable, and like all good things from God, they can become abused. Abuse constitutes sin. Satan hates it when we use the pleasurable things which God has given us appropriately and will use food to try to undermine our relationship with God whenever possible. He did with fruit and Eve, he does it all the time with those trying to lose weight or to avoid unhealthy foods. He has many convinced that chocolate, ice cream or Pringles™ will solve all the problems of the world.

Sugar (and other forms of "junk" food) provides Satan an easy opportunity to do this. Sugar steals and tears down (the health of the body). The food that God created supports and nourishes the body.

Eating (how much and what) is all about self-discipline. Paul explains that we should buffet our bodies and make it our slave (**1 Corinthians 9:27**) so not to be enslaved by any behavior that would interfere with our ministry and purpose God has for us. The Bible gives us many principles that we can learn to judge our eating habits. For example:

✦ Will eating a certain food or drink demonstrate a heart of idolatry? (glorifying self/flesh versus glorifying God?)

✦ Will eating a certain food or drink cause another Christian to stumble?

✦ Will eating a certain food prevent you from eating something healthier?

✦ Does the desire to eat a certain food stem from covetousness?

✦ Does the desire to eat a certain food stem from emotion (anger, depression, boredom, etc.)?

✦ Can you say "no" to certain foods, knowing you can eat them without sin?

✦ Are your food/drink choices and amounts consumed in accordance with God's guidelines for gluttony, addiction, anorexia and bulimia?

✦ Do your food choices demonstrate healthy eating habits for others?

Discipline

Discipline is a requirement for holiness. To *flee from evil* requires discipline. We need to constantly deal with "the evil" in the world and be continually brushing its effects off of us so it does not contaminate us.

When we are convicted that most of the shows on (secular) television do not glorify God and that He does not want us wasting our time watching them, it requires discipline to NOT join in when the rest of the family (who do not share the same revelation) is enjoying it.

It requires discipline to NOT look at the seductive billboards, advertisements, magazine cover, or even people on the street that draw upon the lust of the flesh. This is exactly what they are designed to do – seduce you.

Just as it requires great discipline to fast or live a fasted lifestyle where our food choices consistantly do not solely gratify the flesh (our taste buds), but nourish the body. I thank God that so many of the foods He created for us to eat do taste wonderful!

One time when I was trying to fast, I asked God why it was so hard. He answered plain and simple, "You need discipline!"

To die to the flesh requires discipline. The world

(man) would have us believing many things and it is easy to fall into the trap of man. The world will try to convince us that we need to be married at a certain age, that we need to have children, that we need to go to college, that we need to make a certain amount of money to be successful, that we need to get a new car every two years, that we need prescription drugs, that we need insurance, that we need to be a certain size or shape, that we cannot eat butter because it contains cholesterol, that we need to drink milk to have healthy bones, that we need to have our children vaccinated to protect them from illness, that we should kill unwanted babies and that we should not allow prayer in the schools. These things are all socially acceptable in the world.

Sanctification

Therefore 'Come out from among them and be separate, says the Lord. Do not touch what is unclean, And I will receive you. I will be a Father to you, And you shall be My sons and daughters, Says the LORD Almighty.'
2 Corinthians 6:17-18

Sanctification is the process we go through in order to become more Christ-like, to become a presentable bride. It is the cleansing, purification process of getting rid of all and anything that is unholy and displeasing to God. This is a life-long process. It does not happen in a week or a month or a 40-day fast. It is a lifetime of seeking God, of humbling ourselves and of obedience and maturity. As we grow closer and closer to Him, He will require more and more of us. There must be less of us, so that there can be more of Him in our life.

The sanctification process separates the believer from the world's evil things and ways. This sanctification is God's will for us (as believers) **1 Thessalonians 4:3**, and His purpose for calling us. This process must be learned from God **(4:4)**, as He teaches it by His Word.

Furthermore then we beseech you, brethren, and exhort you by the Lord Jesus, that as ye have received of us how ye ought to walk and to please God, so ye would abound more and more. For ye know what commandments we gave you by the Lord Jesus. For this is the will of God, even your sanctification, that ye should abstain from fornication: That every one of you should know how to possess his vessel in sanctification and honor. **1 Thessalonians 4:1-4**

For they verily for a few days chastened us after their own pleasure; but He for our profit, that we might be partakers of His holiness. Now no chastening for the present seemeth to be joyous, but grievous: nevertheless afterward it yieldeth the peaceable fruit of righteousness unto them which are exercised thereby. Wherefore lift up the hands which hang down, and the feeble knees; And make straight paths for your feet, lest that which is lame be turned out of the way; but let it rather be healed. Follow peace with all men, and holiness, without which no man shall see the Lord: Looking diligently lest any man fail of the grace of God; lest any root of bitterness springing up trouble you, and thereby many be defiled. **Hebrews 12:10-15**

This is a process which must be pursued by the believer, earnestly and undeviatingly. It is an individual, and sometimes lonely pursuit between you and God, in obedience to the Word of God, and of following the example of Christ, in the power of the Holy Spirit. The Holy Spirit is the agent in sanctification, *That I should be the minister of Jesus Christ to the Gentiles, ministering the gospel of God, that the offering up of the Gentiles might be acceptable, being sanctified by the Holy Ghost.* **Romans 15:16**

The Pain of Purification

Purification is the process of sanctification we go

through to be more Christ-like. It is the cleansing and purging of things in our life that God wants us to get rid of. It is usually not pleasant to "go through the fire of purification" (**Zec. 13:9**), but is so necessary as part of the growth in our relationship with Him. God loves analogies. Here are a few:

Cleansing

We all need cleansing. If we are in the world, we are going to get dirty. And as we get dirty, we can't always see the dirt that is on us. Some dirt gets stuck to the under side of our arms, the back side of our legs or ears, and is easy to overlook. Yet, it may be plainly visible to others. Have you ever showered after painting or doing yard work, and found later that you "missed" some areas and thought, "How did I miss that?" It is the same way with with our spiritual walk towards holiness.

In fasting, we need to ask God to reveal to us the "spots" that we cannot see so that we can be totally cleansed.

During a fast it is important to drink lots of water to flush the body of the toxins which have accumulated over the years. When we are not fasting and consuming food on a regular basis, it is actually work for the body to digest that food. The enzymes produced by the pancreas are used as part of the digestive process. This is especially true if we are consuming a lot of processed and refined foods which contain no enzymes. Live enzymes in our food are destroyed by the heat of cooking. Therefore, cooked food contains no enzymes.

Sometimes, when I am in a sarcastic mood, I call it dead food. However, just because a food is cooked does not mean that it has no nutritional value, it is simply less nutritious than it was in it's natural raw form. It is good (if possible) to eat as much raw foods as possible.

This is one of the attributes of juicing. The enzymes in the raw foods help take the burden off of the pancreas (which would otherwise have to produce digestive enzymes) to break down the foods we eat.

A note of interest: Eagles never eat dead food!

My definition of natural:
As created by God... unaltered by man.

In a juice fast, it is best to only consume juice prepared from live fruits and vegetables, this provides a great opportunity for the body to use the enzymes produced by the liver and pancreas for other important housekeeping issues, such as cleaning toxins and debris out of our cells.

Where did the toxins come from? We are surrounded by them in our environment. We absorb industrial waste, herbicides, pesticides, additives and heavy metals from our food (especially meat and dairy products), water, air, cosmetics. etc. In a large survey conducted by the Environmental Protection Agency in 1990, every person tested showed evidence of petrochemical pollution (such as styrene from plastics, xylene from paint and gasoline solvents, benzene from gasoline and toluene) in their tissues. Fat tissues especially readily hold onto these toxins. The world is highly contaminated and as we live in it, some of it simply gets pushed onto us whether we like it or not. (Just as living in the world contaminates us with sin.)

As these toxins are released into the blood stream, they will often create some unpleasant effects which are discussed in a later chapter on Fasting Basics. Drinking lots of water helps speed up the removal of these toxins which helps to lessen their effects in the body. You are likely to notice changes in your body as these toxins move out of their hiding places in our cells and tissues before they are released out of the body. This is a good thing, even though the effects (increased body odor, headaches, muscle aches, etc.) may not be very pleasant.

As I was thinking about this, God reminded me of the spiritual and emotional cleansing which also occurs in fasting. As we are seeking God in fasting, He will reveal toxic things that He wants us to get rid of. We know it needs to come out as it's not good for us. If it stays it could create problems down the road. The problem is that it is uncomfortable to let go. Emotional woundings we have buried need to be dealt with so God can heal the damage they created. God can't get in there and heal us if we have our walls up.

When you fast, drink lots of water, take lots of showers, and bathe yourself in prayer and God's presence so He can take care of you the way He wants to.

Husbands, love your wives, even as Christ also loved the church, and gave Himself for it; That He might sanctify and cleanse it with the washing of water by the

word, That He might present it to himself a glorious church, not having spot, or wrinkle, or any such thing; but that it should be holy and without blemish.
Ephesians 5:26-28

The Fire

Purification in our lives can also be compared to the refining process of metal. The purpose of going "through the fire" is to burn off all the dross, the impurities of silver which are separated out in the melting process, which requires extreme heat. The impurities must be eliminated to make the metal pure, totally refined, just as our impurities must be eliminated to make us pure, Christ-like.

Take away the dross from the silver, and there shall come forth a vessel for the finer. **Proverbs 25:4**

When He has tried me, I shall come forth as refined gold (pure and luminous). **Job 23:10** AMP

For thou, O God, hast proved us: thou hast tried us, as silver is tried. Thou broughtest us into the net; Thou laidst affliction upon our loins. Thou hast caused men to ride over our heads; we went through fire and through water: but Thou broughtest us out into a wealthy place.
Psalm 66:10-12

Jesus spoke of the unquenchable fire which burns the chaff. This is a stalk of grain from which the kernels have been beaten out. It is essentially the remaining unneeded portion of the plant that was commonly burned to dispose of it.

Whose fan is in His hand, and He will thoroughly purge His floor, and gather His wheat into the garner; but He will burn up the chaff with unquenchable fire. **Matthew 3:12**

Therefore as the fire devoureth the stubble, and the flame consumeth the chaff, so their root shall be as rottenness, and their blossom shall go up as dust: because they have cast away the law of the LORD of hosts, and despised the word of the Holy One of Israel. **Isaiah 5:24**

For many of us, this purification process can be a painful and difficult one. This process of "refining" or "going through the fire" is not easy. Fire hurts. You know this if you have ever had a burn, even a small burn from a hot oven or stove. Yet, fire is something we are often attracted to - to it's warmth perhaps, or the intoxicating effect of watching the flames in a fireplace or bonfire.

From a spiritual standpoint, for those who are called (Ephesians 1), there is a deep yearning to grow closer to God, but at the same time, there is resistance. For some, it is the fear of the fire. The fear of the pain to actually go through the fire; fear to let go of the things (deep woundings) deep inside the hear; afraid to have any of them exposed; afraid to have any of them even brought up to the surface from where they are buried because we don't want to be reminded that they are even there, let alone the pain that they caused us. These things, feeling of failure, shame, condemnation, guilt, embarrassment, inadequacies, and other things that have held us in bondage interfere with our relationship with the Father. Christ died for our sins so we could be set free, not hold onto them and continue to live in bondage.

God knows your heart (better than you do). He knows if you are holding back, holding onto things, He knows if your motives are impure. He tells us these things as a cautionary because He is a jealous God, and He must have our entire affection and adoration. He has a heavy hand to punish things like pride and impure motives, especially in His worship.

For the LORD thy God is a consuming fire, even a jealous God. **Deuteronomy 4:24**

God is so merciful. He continually encourages us to repentance, as an inducement to obedience. God will never forsake us, but we must be faithful to Him.

Prepare Yourself as a Bride

The Bible often refers to His church as the bride waiting for her bridegroom (the return of Christ).

And I, John, saw the holy city, New Jerusalem, coming down from God out of heaven, prepared as a bride adorned for her husband. **Revelation 21:2**

And the Spirit and the bride say, Come. And let him that heareth say, Come. And let him that is athirst come. And whosoever will, let him take the water of life freely. **Revelation 22:17**

Just as a bride wants to present herself to her husband in the most pleasing manner as possible, so are we (as individuals making up the church) to be preparing for our bridegroom Christ Jesus.

A bride may spend days and weeks or longer look-ing for the perfect wedding dress, the perfect shoes, flowers, invitations, photographer, etc. She will proba-bly diet months in advance, have her hair and nails professionally done, all to be pleasing to the groom. She may get facials to sluff off dry dead skin cells and remove impurities from her skin so she can look radi-ant on that special day.

God wants us to do the same – and even more, for Him. God is calling us to holiness. He wants us to get rid of all the dead stuff and impurities which contami-nate our lives and our relationship with him. All of our flesh needs to be burned up so all that is left is a pure transformed heart that only reflects Him. We cannot come into His presence in our own righteousness (*all our righteousness is as filthy rags,* **Isaiah 64:6**), but if we are obedient to seek His will and seek to please Him, then our garments will be white and we will be radiant.

*Let us be glad and rejoice, and give honor to him: for the marriage of the Lamb is come, **and his bride hath made herself ready**. And to her was granted that she should be arrayed in fine linen, clean and white: for the fine linen is the righteousness of saints.* **Revelation 19:7-8**

Let thy garments be always white; and let thy head lack no ointment. **Ecclesiastes 9:8**

My heart aches because it *seems* like no one (or few very) is getting ready... no one is preparing for our "big day" when the groom will come for us. No one is fasting, no one cares. Everyone seems to be too caught up with their circumstances and life in this world to realize that we are not ready. The bride is not ready. He could come at any time!!!!

Jesus taught of the need of purity and simplicity as the motive for the bride to fast as he refers to Himself as the Bridegroom.

And Jesus said unto them, Can the children of the bridechamber mourn, as long as the bridegroom is with them? but the days will come, when the bridegroom shall be taken from them, and then shall they fast. **Matthew 9:15**

The following is a moving and interesting prophetic insight from Michal Ann Goll, of Ministry to the Nations, Franklin, TN. She has a tape entitled, "Releasing the Fire Bride!" where she speaks of a 3-week angelic visitation she experienced.

She says, "*I heard Jesus sing to His Father, 'Where is my bride, oh my God?'*" She talks about the importance of a personal relationship with Jesus, "*but do we really know Him? How can we say we know him when we have only shook his hand a few times? Have we really spent enough time with him to claim that we know him?*"

Do we know Jesus as well as we know someone who we would marry or are married to? How much time do we spend with Him compared to someone we are engaged to be married to?

A bride makes preparation in great excitement. We complain and mumble. A bride pours her whole heart into the smallest of details for the cake, the dinner menu, the napkins, her hair, jewelry, dress and shoes. We drag our feet like the Jews in Haggai who were instructed to build the temple for God. They neglected and put off the building of God's house so that they might have time and money for their secular affairs (building their own houses). They desired to be excused from such an expensive piece of work under the pretense that they must provide for their families, and until they have gotten settled in the world, they cannot think of rebuilding the temple.

Sound familiar? God said to them through the prophet Haggai, *Is it time for you, O ye, to dwell in your ceiled houses, and this house lie waste? Now therefore, thus saith the LORD of hosts; Consider your ways. Ye have sown much, and bring in little; ye eat, but ye have not enough; ye drink, but ye are not filled with drink; ye clothe you, but there is none warm; and he that earneth wages earneth wages to put it into a bag with holes. Thus saith the LORD of hosts; Consider your ways.* **Haggai 1:4-7**

There is much we should be doing (now, and not putting off until later) to be preparing for our bridegroom. We are so selfish. We are so caught up in our flesh and the world that we do not even realize our own sinfulness. We do not realize how repulsive our attitudes and ways are to the most high God.

Take ye heed, watch and pray: for ye know not when the time is. For the Son of man is as a man taking a far journey, who left his house, and gave authority to his servants, and to every man his work, and commanded the porter to watch. Watch ye therefore: for ye know not when the master of the house cometh, at even, or at midnight, or at the cock crowing, or in the morning: Lest coming suddenly he find you sleeping. **Mark 13:33-36**

Are we ready? Are you ready? Are you putting off dealing with issues that God is calling you to? Are you serving Him to your full capacity?

From the tape:
"The Lord is requiring us to submit to His flames to become a fire bride. To become a fire bride, fire must consume our chaff. We are forever engraved on the "Lord's Arm." If the bride could only understand that His love is big enough to cover ALL her failings, weaknesses, her needs, all her ailments. He's already made full payment.

As the bride runs to the Lord crying, "HELP ME!", the air fuels the fire, burning the dross off—when she sees this, she cries out all the more, 'MORE FIRE, LORD!'"

For more information on Jim and Michal Ann Goll and Ministries to the Nations, visit http://www.ministrytothenations.org/

Power

Flesh verses Spirit

The battle of flesh versus spirit is an ongoing struggle that we must face everyday as Christians. We are told to die to the flesh – and this is something that must be done daily. We are physical, fleshly human beings.

That the righteousness of the law might be fulfilled in us, who walk not after the flesh, but after the Spirit. For they that are after the flesh do mind the things of the flesh; but they that are after the Spirit the things of the Spirit. For to be carnally minded is death; but to be spiritually minded is life and peace. Because the carnal mind is enmity against God: for it is not subject to the law of God, neither indeed can be. So then they that are in the flesh cannot please God. **Romans 4:8**

Those *that are after the flesh* are under the influence of the flesh, and therefore, cannot be influenced by the Spirit. Sin (intentional repetitive sin, or sin which you have long ignored the Holy Spirits prompting for you to get rid of it) in our life can inhibit the Holy Spirit from working in us. God (in His holiness) cannot be in the presence of sin. "*Do mind*" in this scripture refers to what you give your attention to – your focus. If *the things of the flesh* are the predominating influence (over the things of the Spirit) this will reflect itself in the character of your actions.

There can be only one master. You cannot be on both sides of the fence at the same time. You must be hot or cold. If you are lukewarm, you get spewed!

Whose end is destruction, whose God is their belly, and whose glory is in their shame, who mind earthly things. **Philippians 3:19**

For if ye live after the flesh, ye shall die: but if ye through the Spirit do mortify the deeds of the body, ye shall live. **Romans 8:13**

Strongs Concordance states that "flesh" (*sarx* in the Greek) *denotes mere human nature, the earthly nature of man apart from divine influence, and therefore prone to sin and opposed to God.*

For Christ also hath once suffered for sins, the just for the unjust, that he might bring us to God, being put to death in the flesh, but quickened by the Spirit. **1 Peter 3:18**

But I see another law in my members, warring against the law of my mind, and bringing me into captivity to the law of sin which is in my members. O wretched man that I am! who shall deliver me from the body of this death? I thank God through Jesus Christ our Lord. So then with the mind I myself serve the law of God; but with the flesh the law of sin. **Romans 7:23-25**

Luke 4 talks about Jesus as He was led (by the Holy Spirit) to the wilderness where He was tempted by Satan for 40 days.

And Jesus being full of the Holy Ghost returned from Jordan, and was led by the Spirit into the wilderness, Being forty days tempted of the devil. And in those days he did eat nothing: and when they were ended, he afterward hungered. **Luke 4:1-3**

And when the devil had ended all the temptation, **he departed from him** *for a season. And Jesus returned in the power of the Spirit into Galilee: and there went out a fame of him through all the region round about.* **Luke 4:13-14**

There are **two very important** things in these last two verses. As Christ suppressed the flesh (going 40 days without eating) **Satan departed from Him.** AND Jesus returned from the desert **in the power of the Holy Spirit.**

As the flesh decreases, the Holy Spirit increases. Through the Holy Spirit is where the POWER is. Fasting increases the POWER of the Holy Spirit in us. This is, to me, one of the most important reasons for fasting. Less of me... means more of God! *He must increase, but I must decrease.* **John 3:30**

After Jesus left the desert, this is when He began to teach with authority and power, cast out demons and heal the people. *And they were astonished at his doctrine: for his word was with power.* **Luke 4:32**

Now when the sun was setting, all they that had any sick with divers diseases brought them unto him; and he laid his hands on every one of them, and healed them. **Luke 4:40**

As Christians, meaning we have accepted Christ into our heart as our personal Lord and Savior, we strive to be like Christ. This practice of sanctification is a life-long process which cannot exist without a personal relationship with God. We must spend time with Him daily. We must study daily and know the word. We must have humble and contrite spirits. It involves listening, discernment, obedience and service which are founded in love, not obligation.

Let this mind be in you, which was also in Christ Jesus: Who, being in the form of God, thought it not robbery to be equal with God: But made Himself of no reputation, and took upon Him the form of a servant, and was made in the likeness of men: And being found in fashion as a man, He humbled himself, and became obedient unto death, even the death of the cross. **Philippians 2:5-8**

As we grow in our personal relationship with Jesus, as we start operating in the gifts of the Holy Spirit, as we gain experience that we have learned from, we need to start mentoring other "younger" Christians. Young Christians are highly vulnerable to Satan's schemes and traps. Without proper instruction, many would be lost or greatly hindered in fulfilling the purpose that God has called them for. Just as many of us have had mentors who took us under their wing to teach us, encourage us and guide us, we need to do the same. The process of discipleship and teaching is of the utmost importance and an important way we all need to be serving.

Satan Will Flee From You!

This is a very important aspect to realize not only about fasting, but in general. Scripture is very clear: *Submit yourselves therefore to God. Resist the devil, and he will flee from you.* **James 4:7**

As Christians, Satan will target us. *And the dragon was wroth with the woman, and went to make war with the remnant of her seed, which keep the commandments of God, and have the testimony of Jesus Christ.* **Revelation 12:17**

As Christians, it seems that all of us go through periods of our life where it seems as though Satan simply will not leave us alone. No matter how much we pray and study and try to be obedient, Satan is there at every corner attacking some aspect of your life: Your health, your house, spouse, children, pets, extended family, church, etc. You cry out to God, "How long is this going to last? I can't take it!"

The answer is that it will continue as long as you allow it!

Oftentimes (unknowingly, of course), we are leaving an open invitation for Satan and his army to come in and attack over and over. As soon as you finish fighting one battle, there he is again coming from another direction. This is a good indication that you have left the back door wide open. This means there is a great possibility that there is **something** in your life that is allowing the attacks to continue. Satan can only do to us what God allows him to do (remember Job?) If God is trying to show us something, He may just allow these attacks to continue until we start paying attention.

It is true, sometimes God will allow Satan to attack us for reasons we cannot understand, but this is not God's plans for us. Usually, He is trying to get a message across to us that we need to deal with. He is trying to grow us up, mature us and bring us closer to Him.

What are the open doors? These may be things like:

Unbelief: Weak faith, doubting, etc. Do you believe without a shadow of a doubt that God will provide?

For verily I say unto you, That whosoever shall say unto this mountain, Be thou removed, and be thou cast into the sea; and shall not doubt in his heart, but shall believe that those things which he saith shall come to pass; he shall have whatsoever he saith. Therefore I say unto you, What things soever ye desire, when ye pray, believe that ye receive them, and ye shall have them.
Mark 11:23-24

Self/Focus: Focusing on yourself and your circumstances instead of on God. *Commit to the Lord whatever you do, and your plans will succeed.*
Proverbs 16:3

Unconfessed Sin: Trying to hide or coverup your sins from God. This results in an unclean conscience.

Sin: Unforgiveness, gossip, backstabbing or any other sin that God wants to purge from you. It could be unfaithful tithing, or maybe God wants you to tithe some place other that where you are. It could be disobedience in any form.

Sinful Behavior in Your Household: (Unknown to you) by someone in your household. This could also include pornographic materials hidden away somewhere, liquor in the house if there is someone who struggles with this issue, etc.

Temptation: Struggling with influences of the flesh.

Lack of Spiritual Support: Lack of prayer, praise and worship, thanksgiving, etc. **(Psalm 34)**

There are, of course, many other things, but you can get an idea through these examples. If we can take care of these types of issues, Satan does not have a chance! He must flee.

Resist the devil, and he will flee from you.

This is where God really gets exciting! We need to **USE** the power and authority that God has given us. We need to learn how to pray and we need to start exercising the power that God has given us through the Holy Spirit.

Using the power is sort of like having a car and the keys to it. It doesn't do you much good if you never get in and drive. At first, you may be very nervous and feel like you do not know what you are doing. That is exactly how God wants us, without the pride of thinking we can do things on our own, but to just rely on Him. Sure you may be a little unsteady, and even go off the road a few times, but as long as you keep it in drive, going forward (instead of backsliding) and continue to rely upon God instead of yourself, you will be fine! It is also great to have more experienced Christians ride along with you to act as mentors. (And then, don't forget to serve as a mentor yourself when God calls you!)

The only thing that can stand between you and your relationship with God is you. The only thing that can stand between you and your walk in the power of God is you.

God wants to empower you to do His kingdom work. *But ye shall receive power, after that the Holy Ghost is come upon you: and ye shall be witnesses unto me both in Jerusalem, and in all Judaea, and in Samaria, and unto the uttermost part of the earth.* **Acts 1:8**

People are drawn to power. People are drawn to miracles, and are looking for signs and wonders. This is why people are drawn to psychics, and even the powers of black magic, etc., but this power does not come from or glorify God, it comes from the deceiver, the counterfeit, to lure people away from the truth. True power is in Jesus.

This draw to power is the reason that Jesus did

miracles. He healed people not only because He had mercy and compassion for them, but because it is an effective tool to demonstrate both His power and love. Use of this power is also what empowers us to spread the gospel.

If God is going to give us the power of the Holy Spirit, it only makes sense that we learn how to use it and use it according to how God wants us to use it. He does this through the word, through discernment and other things which we develop when we have a personal intimate relationship with Him. Once we experience the power and the presence of God, it is something that we can only want more of. As we grow in our knowledge of Him, we realize how little we know and how much more there is to know and understand.

Without a solid base in scripture and without spiritual understanding, we simply cannot practice good discernment. When I look back at my life from the spiritual perspective that I have today, I am simply amazed at how many times I "just didn't see it." I was walking around completely blind, and only by the grace of God was not completely destroyed by the enemy (or myself). But, with God, "ignorance" is not a valid "excuse."

My people are destroyed for lack of knowledge: because thou hast rejected knowledge, I will also reject thee, that thou shalt be no priest to me: seeing thou hast forgotten the law of thy God, I will also forget thy children. **Hosea 4:6**

How to Exercise Your Power Over Satan

Aside from "cleaning up your act," there are three specific simple things you can do to use the authority that God has given us through Christ. Satan hates to hear:

1. The name of Jesus.

Simply state the name "Jesus" out loud when you feel the harassment of Satan or his army.

2. References to the blood of Jesus shed on the cross.

Out loud, plead the blood of Jesus over your whole house, your property, everyone in your household (including pets), ungodly things in your house (that you cannot remove) that they do cannot cause harm or be a door for Satan to come in. Plead the blood of Jesus over your vehicles or any other mode of transportation you plan to use, over your place of work, schools your children attend, etc.

3. The quoted Word of God.

It is very powerful to simply read scripture out loud. This is especially good to do if you are not comfortable praying out loud. The Psalms are very good! My favorites include Psalm 34 (for comfort), and 37, 39, 41-42, 44, 57, 91, 109 (for protection and deliverance) and 119 (for keeping your path straight).

Remember Satan cannot read your thoughts like God can, so you need to vocalize these things out loud. It may seem uncomfortable at first, but it will get easier the more you do it (like driving a car). At first you may not *feel* like you have authority, but you can't ride a bike without learning with the training wheels on first. You just have to do it!

Putting on praise music is also helpful, especially in songs which incorporate the Word of God! Turn up the volume and sing your heart out!

Pray also for angels to be sent forth to protect you, your house and family. They will come! I had been praying for angels daily to come to my house to protect and minister to me and after a while, I asked if I could see the angels He had sent for me. Sure enough, a day or so later during prayer at bible study one night at my house, I looked outside and there were angels everywhere! It was amazing! (I don't see them like I do a physical object, I see a glowing of light.) God really does hear our prayers and His angels are indeed there to serve us.

Be aware of what "your weak areas" are. Satan never plays fair. He always goes for the throat! Never let your guard down! And don't be so surprised when the attacks come if you let your guard down.

Other people can only pray for you so much. You and especially the spiritual head of the house need to take authority and pray for protection everyday.

Do not let Satan steal from you what Christ died for! Command Satan to give back what he has stolen and instruct your angels to go bring them back for you!

Take Full Advantage of ALL God Has For You!

Yep, there's more! Power is just one aspect of the

Holy Spirit just waiting for us to start using. Look at all of the other aspects! **Riches, wisdom, strength, honor, glory,** and **blessing.** These are the things that God has waiting for us. Pray for them... and believe!

Behold, I give you the authority to trample on serpents and scorpions, and over all the power of the enemy, and nothing shall by any means hurt you. **Luke 10:19**

Who gave himself for our sins, that he might deliver us from this present evil world, according to the will of God and our Father. **Galatians 1:4**

The Significance of Food

God created food to nourish our bodies. *And God said, Behold, I have given you every herb bearing seed, which is upon the face of all the earth, and every tree, in the which is the fruit of a tree yielding seed; to you it shall be for meat.* **Genesis 1:29**

Imagine how incredible that must have been to have access to the fruit, herbs, seeds and nuts, perfect in form, free of pesticides, chemicals, preservatives, radiation, etc. Just as God always provides all we need, God provided food for the Israelites when they were in the wilderness. *Man did eat angels' food: he sent them meat to the full.* **Psalm 78:25**

Moses called this food of the angels "manna" and described it...*like coriander seed, white; and the taste of it was like wafers made with honey.* **Exodus 16:31**

The Chaldee explains that the manna "*descended from the dwelling of angels. Every one, even the least child in Israel, did eat the bread of the mighty; the weakest stomach could digest it, and yet it was so nourishing that it was strong meat for strong men. And, though the provision was so good, yet they were not stinted, nor ever reduced to short allowance; for he sent them meat*

131

to the full."

When God sent manna to the Israelites for them to eat, He was trying to teach them to trust and rely upon Him. Exodus 16:4 says, *Then the LORD said to Moses, I will rain down bread from heaven for you. The people are to go out each day and gather enough for that day. In this way I will test them and see whether they will follow my instructions.*

The Lord through Moses also instructed them to use up or to share what they did not need, and to not keep it until the next day or it would turn to maggots. God knew what they would do, but He wanted them to see for themselves that they were not trusting Him. Exodus 16:20 says, *However, some of them paid no attention to Moses; they kept part of it until morning, but it was full of maggots and began to smell. So Moses was angry with them.*

They feared they would not have enough, that they would not be satisfied. They were simply not trusting God. Fear causes people to hoard, to be selfish and to eat too much.

Today, in this time of abundance in our country, many people rarely feel hunger. They eat, drink or snack so often where they just don't experience hunger pains very often, if at all. The fear of not being satisfied or not having enough is not trusting God for His provision for us as His children. We need to hold on to our inheritance, to that promise of faith, that even in famine, because of the Lord's faithfulness, we will be satisfied!

He that hath an ear, let him hear what the Spirit saith unto the churches; To him that overcometh will I give to eat of the hidden manna, and will give him a white stone, and in the stone a new name written, which no man knoweth saving he that receiveth it. **Revelation 2:17**

God promises great favor to those that overcome. He says we shall eat of the hidden manna and have the new name, and the white stone. God wants us to now taste of the hidden manna (the influences and comforts of the Spirit of Christ resulting from constant communion with him), coming down from heaven into our soul, from time to time, for its support. He wants us to taste of how saints and angels live in heaven. This is hidden from the rest of the world. Strangers cannot experience this joy; and it is laid up for those in Christ.

This reminds me of the experience of fasting, and especially a prolonged fast. Going without real earthly food for so long truly reveals another spiritual level that is untapped for many, but is available for us now. But God is calling us to come and taste what He has for us!

Corrupted, Distorted, Man...ipulated!

While God created food to be nourishing to our bodies, He also made food delicious and provided us with taste buds, and the sense of smell to enjoy it. The problem is that these fleshly sensations have tended to overrule the principle of simply eating to maintain the health of the body.

Food and our focus on food has become very corrupt. The problems stem from the manipulation (by man) of the perfect, healthy foods God created, the overindulgence in food and the misuse of food.

It is not God's plan that we are to stress over (or think about) our food and what we eat. Jesus said, *Therefore I say unto you, Take no thought for your life, what ye shall eat, or what ye shall drink; nor yet for your body, what ye shall put on. Is not the life more than meat, and the body than raiment?* **Matthew 6:25**

Food is part of the world and has become part of all the things of the world. For example, what's a ballpark without hot dogs, a movie theatre without pop corn, or a carnival or fair without cotton candy and corn dogs? What's Valentine's Day without chocolate? ... and some people even question what's life without chocolate?!

We cannot live without food as it provides the required nutritional and energy needs for the body to function properly. We have no choice, we must eat. But, we do have a choice as to what we eat, how much we eat and why we eat. If we make good choices, we provide optimal nutrition for the body and we can maintain good health as God intended. God created the body to heal itself, but we have a responsibility to take care of the body that God gave us. These are natural laws (created by God). We cannot expect the fulfillment of spiritual laws (God promises to heal us) if we break His natural laws.

For example, if you have fibromyalgia, migraines, allergies or cancer because your body is so toxic with the chemicals from consuming processed and refined food, pop, sugar, etc, topped with cigarettes, medication, pain killers, etc., God may not heal you until you quit consuming these things and get your body cleaned out!

If you have high cholesterol because you are not exercising and are eating a high fat, high sugar diet, God is probably not going to heal you until you change your eating habits. If He does, and you do not correct your habits which caused the problem in the first place, it will quickly return. We always need to search for and address the root of the problem.

We cannot expect the fulfillment of spiritual laws of healing if we break His natural laws of not taking proper care of the body.

Food is also a social thing. It is enjoyable to go out to eat (if you don't eat this way all the time). It is fun to get together with friends to "do lunch," or to have dinner guests over. And almost everyone looks forward to Thanksgiving or Christmas dinner, when friends and family get together. Most parties and many gatherings are surrounded around food or at least include food or dessert from your huge banquets for fund raising, weddings, church pot-blessing to even your weekly Bible study.

Food played an important role in Biblical culture as well at times of celebration and feasts. Jesus sat down to eat a special meal with his 12 closest friends, which we now call The Last Supper, of which we still acknowledge through holy communion.

Apparently, the action of individuals taking the pleasures of eating and drinking too far was a problem in Bible times, too. God accused the people of Jerusalem of behaving like Babylon: *And behold joy and gladness, slaying oxen, and killing sheep, eating flesh, and drinking wine: let us eat and drink; for tomorrow we shall die.* **Isaiah 22:13**

Before the flood, God saw how great the wickedness of the earth had become, *For as in the days that were before the flood they were eating and drinking, marrying and giving in marriage, until the day that Noah entered into the ark.* **Matthew 24:38**

And look at these very important scriptures in Luke: *And as it was in the days of Noe, so shall it be also in the days of the Son of man. They did eat, they drank, they married wives, they were given in marriage, until the day that Noe entered into the ark, and the flood came, and destroyed them all. Likewise also as it was in the days of Lot; they did eat, they drank, they bought, they sold, they planted, they builded; But the same day that Lot went out of Sodom it rained fire and brimstone from heaven, and destroyed them all. Even thus shall it be in the day when the Son of man is revealed.* **Luke 17:26-30**

How are those times any different from what we are experiencing today? People are eating and drinking to satisfy the desires of their flesh, not to meet their body's nutritional needs. I have heard people make statements like, "that health food has no taste - or tastes awful," or "how can you live on that rabbit food?" What a horrible thing to say about the foods that God designed to specifically provide our bodies with the nutrients they need!

Today we have genetically modified foods (man's idea of improving what God created- GMOs or genetically modified organisms), food (and water) contaminated with pesticides, chemicals, hormones, antibiotics, preservatives and who knows what else! We have food that comes in packages with labels listing the dozens of chemical ingredients it contains that it can hardly even be called food. We have food that you can pick up at a drive-through window that will provide your entire day's requirements for sodium and fat in a convenient wrapper so you can eat it while driving down the road.

People are eating and drinking to satisfy their desires of the flesh, not to meet their body's nutritional needs.

God's perfect plan is for us to eat foods the way He created them as much as possible. God created many foods which we can eat right off of the tree or vine. Some foods (squash, potatoes, beans, etc.) do require simple cooking which is fine as it seems this is how God created them. The problem lies with highly processed and refined foods (white sugar, white flour, etc.), stripped of their God-given nutrients, and also genetically altered food. This is not God's perfect plan. God created every species to reproduce after it's own kind. Modifying the genetic material (DNA) by cross transplanting genes from one organism (plant or animal) to another is a serious violation of God's natural order.

And God said, Let the earth bring forth grass, the herb yielding seed, and the fruit tree yielding fruit after his kind, whose seed is in itself, upon the earth: and it was so. And the earth brought forth grass, and herb yielding seed after his kind, and the tree yielding fruit, whose seed was in itself, after his kind: and God saw that it was good. **Genesis 1:11-12**

Comfort Food and Stress

Comfort foods are often those that remind people of the love and care that come from home-cooked meals: apple pie, ice cream, hot soup, turkey and mashed potatoes, macaroni and cheese, hot chocolate, baked apples, chocolate pudding, peanut butter and jelly, etc. Certain foods like cookies, candy and ice cream are associated with happy times during childhood. Comfort food is typically associated with pleasant, peaceful, happy feelings.

Other comfort "snack" foods such as french fries, M&M's, popcorn, chips, chocolate, licorice, are associated with "instant gratification."

Many claim that major traumatic events such as the September 11, 2001 terrorist attack have restored the interest of the people to God. However, the nation's sales of comfort and snack foods increased by almost 15% in the month following the attack (reported by the Associated Press in November 2001). Dieticians and psychologists report that in the month following the attack that people across the country turned to food to deal with the anxiety of the terrorist attacks and anthrax scares.

Surveys by Registered Dieticians show that more people are turning to sugary and fatty foods during times of stress. These are the foods that provide instant gratification, stimulating a release of dopamine or other pleasure-related hormones, momentarily allowing us to forget our trouble. Stress, both emotional and physical, can alter the normal routines or levels of control people have over their lives. It is a well-known fact that most people turn to food when their anxiety level increases due to personal or environmental instability. Because people don't know they are doing it, it is hard to determine to what extent this happens.

Refined Foods - The Big Lie!

As we live our lives, we live here on earth in the world until we die, or Christ returns. We are instructed to live in the world, but be not of the world. (Romans 12:2) The world has deceived us in many ways; food is just one of those ways. We are tricked to believe that if it tastes good, smells good and looks good, then it is OK to eat, right? WRONG! This is the deceit! Refined foods are like sheep in wolve's clothing!

Satan is an adulterator! He falsifies and makes things impure. He is a deceiver and an imitator.

God created perfect whole natural foods.
Man has adulterated and imperfected the food
God created through additions and subtractions.

If it tastes good, we want to eat it, and sometimes we eat and eat and eat. These foods simply do not satisfy us (they are **deceivers**). Our body continues to crave what it is NOT getting, and we just keep eating, for some reason thinking that eventually we will obtain what our body wants. We are believing a lie!

Refined foods are foods that have been altered by man through processing (cooking, preserving, etc.). Refined foods are most of the foods in the center isles of the grocery stores (fresh meat, bakery and produce sections are usually on the perimeters of stores). Refined foods are those that come in a box, bag or some sort of packaging with a label to tell you what they put in it. Processing is done for many commercial reasons such as to extend shelf life and to produce more convenient food (snack foods, breakfast bars or other ready-to-eat foods, frozen dinners, or canned food (don't forget Spam™!), and boxed dehydrated-type foods such as Hamburger Helper™ or scalloped potatoes, etc.

Examples of Unrefined (Real) Foods
All fresh vegetables and greens
All whole grains and cereals
Nuts and Seeds
Legumes
All fresh fruit
Milk (only fresh, unpasteurized)
Raw honey (unpasteurized)

Sugar cane
Fresh maple syrup
Fresh meat, poultry or seafood
Herbs and spices

Examples of Refined Foods (avoid these)
Flour
Cornstarch
White rice
Bread (commercial), crackers, chips
Pasta
Sugar
Corn syrup, fructose, factose, maltose and other
refined sugar forms
Sorbitol, aspartame, Splenda™ (sucralose)
Hydrogenated and partially hydrogenated oils
Soda pop

Because processing removes a great deal of the naturally occurring nutrients, these foods are simply not as healthy as they would be if you were to take the time to prepare them yourself from scratch using wholesome ingredients.

Another HUGE problem is all of the NON-FOOD chemicals added to refined foods to lengthen their shelf life and make them better tasting and more visually appealing (more deceit). Common food additives include preservatives (such as benzoic acid, nitrates, sulfites and MSG), coloring agents (food dyes), taste and odor modifiers, texture modifiers and processing agents. Also found in many processed foods are lead, aluminum, mercury, other toxic metals, and don't forget herbicide residues. Numerous books have been written about the health problems associated with these chemicals.

Next time you go to the market, go to the breakfast aisle. Look at the syrup labels and see how many actually contain maple syrup. Unless the bottle actually says "pure maple syrup," you will see that none of them even contain any maple syrup (only maple flavoring)! When you start reading food labels you will be amazed to see how many foods do not actually contain what you think they should. Another example: pineapple yogurt contains no pineapple, only pineapple flavoring.

Because refined foods do not adequately satisfy our nutritional needs, they are the foods we tend to over eat on. Have you ever over eaten fresh broccoli or apples? I don't expect so, yet, we could pretty easily eat half a bag of chips or half a box of breakfast cereal (I remember one time when I was in high school my younger brother ate a whole box of Life™ cereal. How ironic! There is no "life" in Life™ cereal, which is highly processed!

Have you even eaten a bag of chips or some other snack food and still felt hungry? Refined foods have had almost all the naturally occurring nutrients stripped out in processing. They may taste good, but they do not satisfy our nutritional needs, so we just keep eating until we are stuffed - and yet will crave more!

Fortified foods are a joke (but it's not funny)! They remove 90% of the nutrients in processing and then add back in maybe 7 or 11 out of the 100+ daily essential vitamins and minerals and call it "fortified." Most of the nutritional value that God originally put in those grains has been processed out. **God put those specific nutrients in those foods for a reason; they all work together to form a perfect food.** These nutrients are needed to properly metabolize the whole food.

Everything that God created is perfect!

Everything that man (on his own) tries to create is not. Everything that man alters is somehow compromised from the perfection that God created.

For example, grains contain chromium, a trace mineral which works with insulin to move glucose, which are simple sugars (also found in grains), into our cells to be burned. Most, if not all of the chromium is refined out in the processing of the grain. Chromium is not one of the minerals which is added back in with fortification. So, when we eat refined grain products, the body needs that chromium in order to burn the glucose. So what happens? If there happens to be any chromium in the body (maybe you also ate an apple with your refined grains) it will use that (because the refined grains are broken down more quickly because most of the naturally occurring fiber was also removed). But then, what will the body do about the chromium it needs to metabolize the sugar from the apple? If the cells cannot process the sugar, the body will store it as glycogen and fat. Instead of burning any fat you consumed (did you add butter or milk to your grains?), it will be stored as well. And you all probably know where.

This is the primary reason for weight gain. This is the reason obesity has become such a huge problem in our population. This is also the reason the incidence of Type II (adult-onset) diabetes is climbing at unbelievable levels and why it is occurring in younger and younger individuals - even children!

So instead of eating some commercial cereal that

contains some oats (refined) we need to be eating real oats, like steel cut oats. Not "old fashioned oats", this only cooks up in a few minutes, whereas steel cut oats takes about 30 minutes to cook. Instead of feeding these boxed sugar-coated instant cereals to your kids (or self), you need to be giving them real food that satisfies them and their nutritional needs. If you say, "they won't eat it," then you have two things to work on: teaching your children to respect what you say and what you tell them to do, and retraining their taste buds to appreciate real food. If they don't learn how to eat good food when they are young, how are they supposed to know how to eat when they are older? We need to teach our children to respect and obey us, so they will respect and obey God!

Parents need to set an example for their children in all areas of their life. If you eat garbage, they are going to eat garbage.

Often, the more processing a food goes through, the more expensive it is. Manufactures are making a lot of money distorting the perfect foods that God made for us to eat. Compare the price of potato chips to the price of raw potatoes. Think about how many potatoes you can eat (cost wise) vs. how many potato chips you can eat?

Which would you rather eat for a snack, a chocolate bar or an apple? They will both satisfy your sugar craving. However, the chocolate bar contains about four times more calories than the apple and you will probably still be hungry after you eat it. The sugar in the chocolate bar will be quickly absorbed and peak your energy levels and then fall off making you feel tired. The chocolate bar contains no chromium, fiber or other nutrients, so you will most likely not be able to burn all the calories (from the sugar) so you will probably have to store some of them. The saturated fat in the chocolate bar will go into the circulatory system and then has the risk of getting caught up in the plague buildup of the artery walls, potentially increasing your risk for heart attack or stroke.

The apple contains fiber so will be filling and will satisfy your nutritional requirements to use the food in your body. The fiber helps clean out toxins and debris from your intestinal tract. The fiber allows the sugar to be slowly released into the bloodstream allowing a nice energy boost. The potassium helps regulate your blood pressure and maintain heart health.

Why do we eat so much refined food?

1. **It's often less expensive**
   Raw turbinado sugar costs about $1.30 per lb.
   White, bleached sugar costs about $0.20 per lb.

   Fresh beets cost about $2.50 for 3 medium beets.
   Canned beets (loaded with sodium) cost about $0.45 per 12 oz. can.

2. **More convenient** - precooked, ready-to-eat, drive through pickup or delivery (pizza, etc.) etc.

3. **Deceptive taste** - contains added salt, sugar, fat, etc.

3. **Less filling** - processing removed fiber and nutrients that satisfy our nutritional needs and cravings. These foods provide "empty" calories.

We have been deceived into thinking that because they taste good (or we think it will because it sounded good on the label) and because it was fast and convenient, that the sacrifice to our health was worth it. Satan must laugh and say, "I have them so deceived. Look at how those Christians are treating the temple of their Lord!"

Sugar: The Deceiver

Refined sugar is as much of a deceiver as Satan himself. Sugar tastes good, and makes things much more appealing to us. Eating it doesn't seem to be harmful (in the short term), and in fact can be quite enjoyable.

Sugar is much like a drug. It has addictive properties and numerous adverse side effects. Sugar is not a whole natural food that does not even resemble the original sources that God made – sugar cane and sugar beets. Sugar is highly refined, bleached, fragmented, denatured and completely stripped of all nutrients which were present in its original form. Sugar cane and sugar beets are natural and contain minerals, vitamins, trace elements, enzymes, essential fatty acids, amino acids and very important FIBER. The final processed result is a pure crystallized form of sucrose, a white "pharmaceutically pure" chemical.

Eating sugar actually creates a loss of essential nutrients (such as B vitamins and chromium) which are required to metabolize it in the body. In the processing of raw sugar cane or sugar beets to produce white sugar, over 90% of the naturally-occurring chromium is lost. Chromium is needed for insulin to bring glucose into the cells to be used as fuel. Without chromium, we can't burn these calories, so instead they are converted to fat and stored away.

Compared to sugar, honey (in it's raw form) is practically considered health food because raw honey contains several minerals and nutrients to assist in the body's use of the simple carbohydrate in the form of the naturally occurring sugar in honey, yet the Bible clearly warns us not to eat too much honey.

Hast thou found honey? eat so much as is sufficient for thee, lest thou be filled therewith, and vomit it. **Proverbs 25:16**

It is not good to eat much honey: so for men to search their own glory is not glory. **Proverbs 25:27**

Refined Foods and Acidity

One little-known problem that results from a diet high in refined foods is the negative effect these foods have on the pH of the body. The ideal pH for the body is 7.4 - 7.6, which is slightly alkaline (7.0 is neutral). When God designed the body, He created it to ensure that the blood (which God calls the life flow) is maintained at 7.4 - 7.6. If the pH starts dropping, becoming too acidic, it will use the available buffers in the body to counter the acidity and raise the pH to its needed level. The buffers in the body are the alkaline minerals such as calcium, magnesium, phosphorus, etc. The body stores these minerals in our bones. So guess what happens if the body continually has to take minerals out of our bones to neutralize the blood? Brittle bones, also known as, osteoporosis!

Other symptoms of excess acidity include:

Headaches	Fatigue/low energy
Weight problems	Suppressed immunity
Urinary tract infections	Unexplained achiness
Vaginal/Rectal itch	Candida
Diarrhea/constipation	Irritability
Allergies	Blood sugar problems
Cancer	Infections

A suppressed immune system cannot maintain the optimal health of the body for a prolonged period of time. Cancerous cells, parasites, fungus (including candida) or other invaders are simply going to take over and cause problems.

The effect a food has on the body is based upon the amount of sugar, protein and minerals it contains. Sugar and protein are very acid forming. Minerals are more alkaline forming.

The more refined and processed a food, the more acidic it becomes. As a food loses its mineral content, it becomes more acidic.

Here are some examples of foods and how (in quantities of one oz.) they relatively affect the pH of the body. The higher the number, the more alkaline; zero (0) is neutral and the negative numbers are relative acidity values accordingly. (Young)

The Best Alkaline (+) Foods:

Lecithin (soy) . . . . +38
Wheat grass . . . . +34
Chlorella . . . . +33
Cucumbers (fresh) . . . . +31
Soy sprouts . . . . +30
Alfalfa grass . . . . +29
Barley grass . . . . +28
Radishes (red) . . . . +28
Soy nuts (soaked, air dried) . . . . . +27
Cayenne pepper . . . . +19
Avocado . . . . +16
Eggplant . . . . +15
Tomatoes . . . . +14
Cabbage . . . . +14
Celery . . . . +13
Garlic . . . . +13
Beans (white, lima) . . . . +13
Spinach . . . . +8-13
Soybeans (fresh) . . . . +12
Beets (fresh) . . . . +12
Green beans . . . . +11
Lemons . . . . +11
Carrots . . . . +10
Turnips . . . . +8
Limes . . . . +8
Horse radish . . . . +7
Red Cabbage . . . . +6
Zucchini . . . . +6
Peas (fresh) . . . . +5
Kolrabi . . . . +5
Flax seed . . . . +4
Almonds . . . . +4

Cabbage, white . . . . +3
Cauliflower . . . . +3
Tofu . . . . +3
Potatoes . . . . +2
Lentils . . . . +1
Water . . . . Neutral (0)

The Worst Acidic (-) Foods:

Hard Liquor . . . . -29 to -39
Pork . . . . -38
Beef/Veal . . . . -35
Fruit juice (sugar sweetened) . . . . -33
Beer . . . . -27
Black tea . . . . -27
Artificial sweeteners . . . . -26
Coffee . . . . -25
    (even higher with added sugar)
Eggs . . . . -18 to -22
Chicken . . . . -18 to -22
Mustard . . . . -19
Sugar (white) . . . . -18
Cheese . . . . -18
Peanuts, pecans, pistachios . . . . -13
Mayonnaise . . . . -13
Ketchup . . . . -12
(note the comparison to fresh tomatoes as a result of refining and addition of sugar)
Brown rice . . . . -12
White Bread . . . . -10 to -13
Turbinado (raw) sugar . . . . -10
Fructose (fruit sugar) . . . . -10
Honey . . . . -7
Whole grain bread . . . . -4

Note that artificial sweeteners are even more acidic than white sugar. Note that honey (a natural food created by God) which contains minerals, is only slightly acidic, because although it contains natural sugar it also contains minerals, vitamins and other components to help digest it. Refined white sugar and artificial sweeteners contain no minerals or nutrients to speak of.

Fruit: Fresh fruits are slightly acidic because they do contain natural sugars. Note the drastic change to very acidic when processed sugar is added.

Pineapple	-12
Banana (ripe)	-10
Orange, peach, mango, apricot	-9
Cranberries	-7
Raspberries, blueberries	-5
Strawberries, dates	-4
Cantaloupe, grapefruit	-2
Watermelon	-1
Fruit juice (natural)	-9
Fruit juice (sugar sweetened)	-33

Fat: Most fats are relatively neutral or slightly acidic.

Margarine (remember is more processed)	-8
Cream	-4
Butter	-3
Olive oil	-1

Fasting Increases the Acidity of the Body!

Acidity of foods is a very important thing to take note of while you are fasting. Fasting increases the acidity of the body because of the flushing out of toxins from within our cells. While this is a good and important thing, we need to be careful not to allow the body to develop severe mineral deficiencies at this time.

Note the acidity of fruit juices compared to the acidity of vegetable juices. It is important to have a balance of fruit and vegetable juices when you fast so that you do not further increase the acidity of the body at this time.

Fat-Free Foods: More Deception

When fat free foods first came out I thought it was great! Now we could eat all kinds of foods without having to worry about the fat... or could we?

Here is some information you may find interesting. Fat contains all kinds of flavor, so when it is removed, the manufacturers found that to make the product still taste good, they had to add more sugar or sodium. Be very careful when considering products which are "Fat Free," they often have all sorts of other ingredients added for whatever reason.

Also, without the fat, foods tend to be less filling, so it is easy to eat more, resulting in an intake of more calories than you would have consumed if you had been eating the original. All excess calories are stored as fat, so it doesn't necessarily matter what kind of calories they were.

Fat free foods have a higher glycemic index rating

meaning they have a greater effect on our blood sugar and release of insulin. (The higher the rating, the greater the effect. Pure sugar receives a rating of 100, which is the highest rating.) Many fat free foods can create the same sugar highs and lows which could in the long run be just as detrimental to one's health as the original fat-containing food.

Ice cream is a good example. Fat-free ice cream contains a large amount of sugar which is quickly assimilated into the bloodstream causing a spike in the blood sugar. The sugar in regular ice cream is assimilated a little more slowly because of the fat; however, this fat is largely saturated and will negatively effect your cholesterol levels (and probably your weight as well). In the long run, however, the spiked sugar levels (from the fat-free ice cream) can also affect your triglyceride and cholesterol levels. It's better to eat plain unsweetened yogurt with natural chopped fruit added or just eat an apple (or other nutritious natural food choice)!

Deception, Deception...

Have you ever headed for a breakfast buffet, thinking you are are just going to grab a few pieces of fruit? But, as you were walking through the line, you saw they had bagels (that would be good toasted) and can't forget the cream cheese, and a little bit further... look, fresh waffles! ...which you could put your fresh fruit on! and just a little bit of natural maple syrup or whipped cream. It is so easy to be tempted!

I avoid buffets for exactly this reason! *"Give no place to the enemy!"* It's sort of like going to the grocery store because you are out of laundry soap and carrots.

Going through the produce section is not too difficult, and it is usually close to the door. But, then you have to go all the way to the back of the store for the laundry soap and you pass by the deli section (with all the great imported cheeses and dips) and the bakery section (close your eyes in this area), the dairy section (*look, they have egg nog, must be getting close to the holidays*), the frozen foods section (*where you see your favorite brand of pizzas are on sale and those are always good to have on hand when you don't feel like cooking*) and a few other miscellaneous aisles, where you see a few sale signs to go investigate. So you get to the check out and, oh wait, you forgot the laundry soap. So you go back to get the soap, pick up some crackers for the cheese you picked out, get back to the checkout and the total bill is $42.00 (and you came in for two things).

We may not realize it, but stores are specially designed to do exactly this - increase what we buy and the money we spend. Impulse items are strategically placed where we will see them on the most commonly walked areas that will entice us to buy them. Notice how they put the dairy section in the area furthest away from the door. This is because most people have milk on their list, and will therefore, have to go all the way through the store, even if they only need milk. How many times do you go to the store and leave with just milk?

Not only the positioning of the products, but the packaging is also designed to make the product more appealing. Notice how manufactures started putting "FAT

FREE" on everything, even if it never contained fat in the first place.

We need to stop falling for and believing every advertising and marketing gimmick that is set before us. We need to wake up and starting seeking the Word of God for counsel instead of following along with whatever else the rest of the world is doing.

And be not conformed to this world: but be ye transformed by the renewing of your mind, that ye may prove what is that good, and acceptable, and perfect, will of God. **Romans 12:2**

Just as we need to **RE-TRAIN** our taste buds to appreciate REAL food, instead of all the food that man has altered, we need to purify our minds from how the world has deceived us:

✦ You do not need have the TV on every night, or at all.

✦ You do not need pornography and sex toys to have a satisfying intimate, sexual relationship with your spouse.

✦ You do not need drugs to be healthy.

✦ You do not need drugs to be pain free.

✦ You do not need alcohol to relax you.

✦ You do not need to practice shady business practices and take advantage of people to make a good living.

✦ You do not need to go to college to make a good income and be respected.

✦ You do not need to wear brand names to impress anyone.

✦ You do not need to get caught to be guilty of something.

✦ You do not need to file a law suit to vindicate yourself.

✦ You do not need drugs, surgery or anything else you may hear in a hospital or doctor's office to restore your health (unless God tells you otherwise).

The body can (and will) heal itself of just about anything, even cancer, if given the support it needs to do the work it was created to do.

Why are we so sick? We eat the foods we enjoy, not the ones that support the nutritional needs of the body!

The Choice is Yours!

Health authorities now attribute 75% of our degenerative diseases to be caused by our own lifestyle practices. This refers to our:

DIET: The things we eat (or don't) and drink which cause nutritional deficiencies, excess fat (but insufficient essential fatty acids), excess sugar, inadequate fiber and minerals, etc.

TOXIN EXPOSURE: Nitrates, saccharin, aspartame (Nutri-sweet™, Sweet and Low™), tobacco, pesticides, asbestos, carcinogens created from microwave oven use and even UV rays.

STRESS: Emotional or physical

If your hand hurts because you are holding it on a hot stove burner, you should remove it, right? So if something you are doing is causing the cancerous cells in your body to overrule your immune system and spread uncontrollably, you should remove whatever that is, right?

When we remove the cause, the body is then able to heal itself. It still may hurt for a while after you remove it from the burner, but the healing process cannot begin until you do so. The longer you leave it on the burner, the more damage will be done, but it will eventually heal. This has been proven in cancer patients thousands of times.

The problem lies when the individual does not want to correct or give up the cause. People don't want to give up their diet cola, their pop, chips, bacon, hot dogs, pizza, ice cream, sweets, coffee, fast food, cigarettes, bourbon, beer, diet foods, sugar, bronzed skin, etc.

What God says about our lifestyles in His word is Be ye holy, as I am holy **(1 Peter 1:16).**

If you don't know what it is that is causing the problem, pray and ask God. He will reveal it, but then you will be held accountable to remove it. AND, it may be ALL these things in combination over the years have just plain wore out the body and you have your work cut out for you. You may need to go on a strict diet of fruits and vegetables (organic, if possible) for the next year or so to nourish the body back to health. Yes, it may be very hard. But it can be done; People do it and are healed all the time. (Doctor's usually call this healing remission or a misdiagnosis.)

If it is stress (allowing your circumstances to distract you from your focus on God) that is causing your health problems, you may need to make some changes (find a new job, sort out some family problems, let go of some past hurts, etc.). Yes, this can be painful to do. God can't heal those wounds unless you let Him. Remember that you can't run from God, you need to confront things that are interfering with your relationship with Him.

Health problems can and do result from disobedience (Deuteronomy 28: 22, 27). The medical establishment (representing man and the "world") currently approves of three cancer therapies, none of which do anything about the cause of the cancer.

1. Radiation - Burn it
2. Chemotherapy - Poison it
3. Surgery - Cut it out

The logical way to fight cancer or any illness is to support the immune system and remove the cause. If you repent and ask God to reveal to you what you need to do to be healed, He will reveal it to you! If you are obedient, He will bless you! This is one of the most basic principles in the Bible. If we are obedient, He will bless us. (Deuteronomy 28:1-14) Too often we want the blessing, but are not willing to do our part. We will even go through radiation, chemotherapy and surgery to go around God. He can't bless us if we are not in His will. That's just not how He works!

Overeating, Gluttony

The sin of indulgence of the appetite in eating and drinking is mentioned several times in the Bible. *When thou sit to eat with a ruler, consider diligently what is before thee: And put a knife to thy throat, if thou be a man given to appetite. Be not desirous of his dainties: for they are deceitful meat* (**Proverbs 23:1-3**). We must restrain ourselves into moderation, from all excess.

Be not among winebibbers; among riotous eaters of flesh: For the drunkard and the glutton shall come to poverty: and drowsiness shall clothe a man with rags. **Proverbs 23:20-21**

The reason we eat has become very corrupt. Yes, food can and should be enjoyed. The problem stems from the overindulgence and misuse of it. Too many people are living to eat, instead of eating to live.

Instead of eating when we are hungry and stopping when we are full, we stuff ourselves to the point of discomfort and eat when we are bored, depressed, stressed, lonely, and even out of simple habit. Some people are just addicted to food.

Many times, overeating is fear-based. Many people

have deep-rooted fears resulting from unmet needs from some time in their life. These unmet needs often stem from childhood and often involve unhealed woundings involving parents (lack of attention and neglect, abuse, abandonment issues or death, etc.), also broken hearts, unmet dreams, etc. Food becomes a temporary (but false) source of gratification, instead of turning to God and allowing Him to free you from these burdens.

Eating disorders are rampant today, yet far too little discussed. Most people do not seem to realize that misuse of food IS sin. Someone once said to me, "*They* (I assume she meant the church) *have taken away our cigarettes, drugs, alcohol, sex* (I assume she meant extramarital)... *food is the only thing we have left!*"

I am not sure why so many think that when I talk to them about Biblical nutrition, that I am going to tell them they can't or won't enjoy eating any more. The foods that God made are absolutely delicious! Satan has simply distorted the minds of many into thinking otherwise.

Anorexia (self-starvation, denial of food, etc.) and bulimia, uncontrolled eating (binging), following by purging are usually both rooted in unworthiness, self-rejection and fear (fear of rejection, fear of abandonment, etc.). bulimia is later compounded by gluttony and idolatry (using food for comfort instead of God).

Did you know that these disorders are actually "popular" in jr. high and high school today? I was only 15 or 16 years old when I became bulimic. This pattern quickly became a stronghold in my life which I battled with for almost 20 years. When I was saved at age 31, it was by sheer disciple that I overcame. But, when the Holy Spirit was able to operate in my life a few years later, it was simply no longer a struggle. God had to teach me how to eat! Hallelujah!

Later, as God began to teach me about fasting and a fasted lifestyle, I believe that this completely and permanently destroyed any remaining traces of this stronghold in my life. My focus became centered upon Him and not on my self or upon food.

A few months after moving from southern California to Minnesota, I received a phone call that a friend of mine was in the hospital. I was one of the few she would talk to about her eating disorder. We met at Bible study at church. She was a mighty woman of God, spirit-filled, yet weighted perhaps 60lbs on her 5' 8" frame. I tried to talk to her on the phone but she was too weak. She died the next day... on my birthday. She was 23 years old.

I knew that God would turn that around for good. And He has. For many years, even after I was delivered, I never spoke about my eating disorder with anybody. But today, I will no longer hide in shame for the years I was tormented by Satan. I AM a new person in Christ! I will talk openly to anyone who will listen. I know this is one reason it has been so difficult to get this book to press as the bulk of it was written in the fall of 2001. But... persistence wears out resistance!

(Isn't it interesting that God gave me the name for this book back in 2001, "Spewed"... I had no idea then that He would have me writing about my bulimia in this book! God can always take what the enemy meant for bad and turn it into good!)

All that time in fasting and prayer has allowed God to reveal to me the roots of the health problems and strongholds in my life. This allowed the wounds (many from early childhood) which opened the door for the enemy to operate in my life to be healed (and sealed).

God has taught me how to eat! How to eat to live and NOT to live to eat. He has taught me how to see myself as HE sees me! Any of our thoughts (especially about ourself) that do not line up with HIS thoughts open the door for the enemy to attack us!!!! We need to identify the lies we have been believing and come into the truth! AMEN!

This book is POWERFUL because fasting is POWERFUL! I know that prayer and fasting can help reveal any stronghold (and the roots of them) in your life... food related or not.

Other addictions (alcohol, drugs, gambling, sex, etc.) can also stem from a fear-based behavior pattern (fear of rejection, fear of abandonment, fear of man - the opinion of others, etc.).

From time to time we perhaps all have done this: Turn to food (or alcohol, etc.) for the wrong reason. None-the-less, it is wrong and can be a dangerous trap (of Satan) to fall into. Looking in the refrigerator for comfort, to calm down after a stressful day, to raise our spirits if we feel depressed or bored, or to eat at any other time than when you feel hungry or when the body has certain nutritional needs is not good. It is sinful to look to *anything* other than God for our hope and solutions.

Obsession with food is just as detestable to God as alcoholism, drug addiction, pornography, lying, or any

other sin is to Him. Food addictions may be more difficult to deal with because we have to eat to survive and
temptation is all around us all the time, unlike alcohol
or drugs, which can be given up completely.

John 6:41 states, *I am the bread which came
down from heaven.* Verse 58 continues, *he that
eateth of this bread shall live for ever.*

He reminds them of the Israelites in the desert and
their obsession with what they would eat. *This is that
bread which came down from heaven: not as your
fathers did eat manna and are dead* (**John 6:58**). *It is
the spirit that quickeneth; the flesh profiteth nothing: the
words that I speak unto you, they are spirit, and they
are life* (**John 6:63**). It is clear that our focus is not to
be on fleshly concerns – as God will provide. We are to
place our focus on things of the spirit.

---

*Just because everyone else is doing it...
doesn't make it OK with God!*

It is estimated that over 60% of Americans are above
their ideal weight. Obesity, defined as weighing over 20%
of your ideal weight, is a major nutritional concern in
America today, reaching epidemic status. More than
one-third of all adults and one in five children are obese.
Each year, obesity causes at least 300,000 deaths in the
U.S. and costs the country more than $139 billion on
healthcare, diets and diet-related products – and we are
still fat. We are even slower to learn than the Israelites!

While overeating is not the only reason for weight problems, it certainly plays a significant role. Many people take great pleasure in simply stuffing themselves at mealtime, going to all-you-can-eat buffets for one helping after another or eating an entire bag of chips or cookies in one sitting. I can't picture Jesus at a buffet over-indulging or even eating at a fast food place (He may go there to reach out to the lost, but not to eat). If we claim we are Christians, how is this behavior for us Christ-like?

And he said to them all, If any man will come after me, let him deny himself, and take up his cross daily, and follow me. **Luke 9:23**

Food, as it is needed to sustain life, is a very difficult thing for us as humans to give up. But if we realize that Christ is our bread of life, and demonstrate this belief in faith by not eating, we can experience the power of fasting and the truth of God's word. Jesus said: *I am the living bread which came down from heaven: if any man eat of this bread, he shall live for ever: and the bread that I will give is my flesh, which I will give for the life of the world.* **John 6:51**

The reason for fasting is not for weight control, but did you realize that if you fasted for one day a week for a year, you would be consuming approximately 106,000 fewer calories? One pound is equivalent to 3,500 calories, so there is potential to lose over 30 pounds over a year's time exists (providing you don't make up for the loss on the other days).

The spiritual benefits of fasting are so awesome –

allowing such a personal intimacy with God so He can really work in your life. The weight-control benefits are just part of the built-in wisdom of our all-knowing Lord.

Fast Food, Gluttony and Sin?

An interesting article, *Is eating on the run as big a sin as gluttony?* by Janet Street-Porter, author of *Coast To Coast*, examines common eating habits.

She points out "*Italy's Catholic bishops declare that fast food is anti-Catholic and that the act of eating it undermines fundamental Christian values* and states that *the humble hamburger is lacking the community spirit of sharing. It seems that eating on the run is as big a sin as gluttony (eating too much)."*

"*Fast food too often means eating quickly so you can rush off and do other things....Let us not confuse the consumption of fast food with the experience of eating a meal together with friends or family. While the popularity of cooking programs increases on television, our cooking skills atrophy and sales of ready-cooked meals soar. The time when the family shares a meal at the end of each day is ending. No one seems willing to take the time to prepare healthy meals for their family... Our poor health and weight problems show it."*

Everyone is so busy...no one has time to cook, to spend quality time with their family, to pray, to go to church. The world is doing a good job of sidetracking us off of our focus on God.

If Satan doesn't make us bad, he'll make us busy!

Food Choices

A major reason for health problems and excess weight is poor food choices and malnutrition. We eat too much processed food with low nutrient value – "junk food." These foods literally provide "empty calories" – little or no nutritional value other than the calories they provide. But, if we cannot use these calories, they are readily stored as fat. Refined foods lack the nutrients required for efficient energy production and tremendously increase the body's requirement for them. Unrefined foods (the way God made them!) naturally contain these nutrients (B Vitamins, Vitamin C, chromium, magnesium, manganese and other trace minerals), but they are lost in processing.

Family and Fellowship

It is the responsibility of the parents, and especially mothers, to cook and prepare love-filled meals for the family to sit down together and enjoy. This not only is a time where the family's nutritional needs can be met, but is an important time of fellowship and of ministering to one another and a time to pray together.

This is also an important time for the children to spend time in the kitchen before and after the meal in learning how to cook and other important skills; in learning how to help serve the family. etc. It is a sad thing when I hear a teenaged girl say, "I don't know how to cook." I know I was in the kitchen cooking before I was 10 and now people ask me all the time how I learned to cook so well. Thanks Mom!

The Basics of Fasting

Fasting is about sacrifice - unto God. Fasting is a serious commitment between you and God.

Receiving God's best blessing from a fast requires solid commitment to the promises you make to Him. Arranging special time each day with God is absolutely crucial. You must devote yourself to seeking God's face, even (and especially) during those times in which you feel weak, vulnerable, or irritable. Read His Word and pray during mealtimes instead of eating. Meditate on Him when you awake in the night. Sing praises to Him. Focus on your Heavenly Father and make every act one of praise and worship. God will enable you to experience His command to "pray without ceasing" as you seek His presence.

The enemy will target you because he knows that fasting is a powerful Christian discipline. Satan wants you to focus on your flesh and other things of the world where he rules. He certainly does not want you to experience the Power of the Holy Spirit! You must shield yourself from these attacks with the Armor of God and the word of God. Stay in prayer.

Satan will do everything he can to pull you away from your prayer and Bible reading time. When you feel the enemy trying to discourage you in any way, immediately go to God in prayer and ask Him to strengthen you in the face of difficulties and temptations.

Reasons To Fast

This book is about fasting with a spiritual purpose, not designed with a physical purpose such as for weight loss or cleansing. True spiritual fasting focuses on God.

Your fast should be centered on Him, and in this your attitudes, actions, motives, desires, and words should be centered on His as well. This can only take place if God and His Holy Spirit are at the center of our attention. Confession and repentance from your sins as the Holy Spirit brings them to your attention allows a cleansing and healing of our hearts. This must be done so that we can focus on God and God alone so that your prayers may be powerful and effective.

Fasting is about FREEDOM!

In Luke, following his 40-day fast Jesus said, *The Spirit of the Lord is upon me, because he hath anointed me to preach the gospel to the poor; he hath sent me to* **heal the brokenhearted**, *to preach deliverance to the captives, and recovering of sight to the blind, to* **set at liberty them that are bruised**. **Luke 4:18**

We must be FREED from the things that are interfering with our relationship with God and our Lord Jesus! These interferences come from broken hearts, unforgiveness, bitterness, abuse, insecurities, health problems, bondages to sin and other things that cause us to put up walls. You may not even know these things (walls) are there, and that's why we fast. Through fasting, as the Holy Spirit rises up (as we push down our flesh) these things will be revealed so that we can deal with them so that God can then heal those deep woundings. This is what God wants! He wants to heal us so that intimacy can be restored.

A renewed closeness with God and a greater sensitivity to spiritual things are usually the results of a fast. Do not be disappointed if you do not have a "mountaintop experience," as some have. Many people who have successfully completed extended fasts tell of feeling a nearness to God that they have never before known, but others who have honestly sought His face report no particular outward results at all. For others, their fast was physically, emotionally, and spiritually grueling, but they knew they had been called by God to fast, and they completed the fast unto Him as an act of worship; God will honor that commitment. We do not always realize the things that have gone on in a spiritual sense - this does not make the fast less powerful.

Your motive in fasting must be to glorify God. When your motives are right, God will honor your seeking heart and bless your time with Him in a very special way.

1. Show God your love for Him. Make your fast an act of worship, an act of love.

2. Obedience/Repentance. We all have sin.
I humbled my soul with fasting; and my prayer returned into mine own bosom. **Psalm 35:13**

169

When I wept, and chastened my soul with fasting, that was to my reproach. **Psalm 69:10**

3. Power. The more we "push down" the desires of the flesh, the more the Spirit can rise up in its power to work in us. Increase your sensitivity to the Holy Spirit. Fasting stirs up power from God within us to break bondages. Fasting allows God to free us from whatever we need to be freed from!

4. Revival. Personal revival, revival for your church, community, nation, for the world and for the fulfillment of the Great Commission.

5. Personal needs. God wants to bless us, but sometimes there are things that we need to do (or stop doing, etc.) before God can bless us. It is a time of waiting on God, waiting to hear from God, of humbling and repentance.

6. Mourning for self or others
There was great mourning among the Jews, and fasting, and weeping, and wailing; and many lay in sackcloth and ashes. **Esther 4:3**

7. Interceding and deliverance for you, your loved ones, your friends, your church, your pastor, your community, your nation, and the world.
Howbeit this kind goeth not out but by prayer and fasting. **Matthew 17:21**

Use fasting to strengthen your spiritual muscles. Fine tune your ability to "die to self" and your physical needs and desires.

Christian fasting is very different from Hindu fasting which focuses on the self and tries to get something for a perceived sacrifice. Christian fasting focuses on God. The results are spiritual that glorify God, both in the person who fasts and others for whom we fast and pray for.

Isaiah 58:6-8 lists warnings as well as positive results that can occur when we submit ourselves to the discipline of fasting. It is as important to learn from this passage the kinds of fasts that do not please God as it is to understand those fasts He desires. God's people in Isaiah's day had been fasting, but without results. They ignored the way fasting should change their lives and treated it as an empty ritual. Anyone can stop eating and say they are fasting, but this is not an act of worship or a spiritual experience unless God is the focus of the fast. It is not a fast if you just didn't have time to eat all day. Fasting is not an afterthought. Fasting is preplanned, prayed about before and during and is purposefully God centered. You need to take time – MUCH time, out of your day to pray and spend time with God. Don't choose your fasting days on days which you are too busy to eat – this defeats the whole purpose and God will not be glorified.

The purpose of all worship, including fasting, is to prepare our hearts and to glorify God. We worship not to gratify ourselves, but to humble ourselves, change our heart, repent and to magnify God!

God wants us to fast, but also to expand fasting through our actions into our everyday lives. We are to practice discipline and die to the flesh daily. Through the prophet Joel, God called His people to *Turn to Me with all your heart, with fasting* (**Joel 2:12**). We may assume that Isaiah is communicating God's desire that fasting be continued, and that its effects be evidenced beyond the mere private and personal.

Isaiah 58 shows us nine examples of what God expects out of our fasting. These examples are not the only kinds of fasts available and they are **not** to be considered as different fasts. One fast could technically serve all points. There is also not only one type of fast for a particular problem. These are just examples to use and adjust to your own particular needs and desires as you seek to grow closer to God.

1. *To loose the bands of wickedness* (Isaiah 58:6). To free ourselves and others from yokes and strongholds to sin, oppression, addictions, etc.

2. *To undo the heavy burdens* (Isaiah 58:6). To solve problems, inviting the Holy Spirit's aid in lifting loads and tearing down walls that keep ourselves and our loved ones from walking joyfully with the Lord.

3. To *let the oppressed* (physically and spiritually) *go free* (Isaiah 58:6). This is referring to revival and soul winning, to free people everywhere enslaved by sin and to pray to be used of God to bring people out of darkness into the light.

4. To *break every yoke* (Isaiah 58:6), conquering the mental and emotional problems that would control our lives, and return the control to the Lord.

5. To *share our bread with the hungry and to care for the poor* (Isaiah 58:7). To meet the humanitarian needs of others, sometimes called the **Widow's Fast.**

6. To allow **God's *light to break forth like the morning* (Isaiah 58:8)**, bringing clearer perspective and insight as we make crucial decisions.

7. So *thine health shall spring forth* (Isaiah 58:8) sanctification and physical healing.

8. That *your righteousness shall go before you* (Isaiah 58:8), that our testimonies and influence for Jesus will be enhanced before others.

9. That *the glory of the Lord to be their reward* (Isaiah 58:8) for favor and protection against the enemy.

Ways To Fast

The following four kinds of fasts are simply guide-lines you may follow. These can be modified as God directs you.

1. Normal Fast

This fast abstains from food for a definite period during which you ingest only liquids (water and/or juice). The duration can be of any length: one day, three days, one week, 21 days, one month or 40 days. Extreme care should be taken with longer fasts.

2. Absolute Fast

This fast obstains from food and water for a short time - no longer than three days. Moses, Elijah and Jesus all fasted in this way for 40 days; but this would kill anyone without supernatural intervention, and should not be attempted today. Be sure to test the spir-it that tries to talk you into a 40-day fast. Most people have difficulty going one day without water.

3. Partial Fast

This fast omits certain foods (such as sweets, pop coffee, etc.) or is on a schedule that includes limited eating. It may consist of omitting one meal a day for any duration of time.

Eating only fresh vegetables (sometimes called a Daniel Fast) is a good partial fast. Daniel 10:3 discuss-es the three-week period in which he abstained from delicacies (such as desserts and sweets), meat and wine.

God instructed Ezekiel to eat a diet of bread)and gave him the ingredients for the bread) and water. see appendix on page 261.

John Wesley ate only bread (whole grain) and water for many days. Elijah practiced partial fasts at least twice. John the Baptist also participated in partial fasts.

Those individuals who have hypoglycemia or other health problems might consider this kind of fast.

Fasting Variations

John Wesley, the founder of the Methodist denomination, fasted every Wednesday and Friday and required all of his clergy to do the same. Effective ministers of God from the apostle Paul to Martin Luther to John Calvin made it a continual part of their walks with God.

There is really no such thing as one "right" way to fast. Fasting is about the condition of the heart, not the number of days or what you are obstaining from.

You can fast one meal, one day, one week, two weeks. You can fast from all sweets and refined foods, for one day, one week, two weeks, etc. As you start praying about fasting and asking God what He would have you do to grow closer to Him and to control your flesh, you may even feel convicted to get rid of these things completely from your diet.

I had some "favorite" snacks that I used to enjoy frequently that I strongly felt convicted that I needed to simply give up, so I had to. You may feel this about smoking, hard alcohol, wine, beer, pop, sugar, coffee, chocolate, refined foods, etc. It is not that all these things are bad in themselves (well, actually they *are*, but God does not forbid us from them), it is how we view them. God wants us to be free of any and all strongholds in our life. If there is <u>anything</u> that may interfere with your relationship and intimacy with God, you had better get rid of it!

All things are lawful unto me, but all things are not expedient: all things are lawful for me, but I will not be brought under the power of any. **1 Corinthians 6:12**

It is good to start slowly. Don't start out with an extended fast. Instead, fast for one meal a day, then one day a week, then three days, and then one week a month. Build up your spiritual muscles so that you will be prepared in a period of several months or year to fast for an extended 40-day period.

Whatever type of fast you choose, be sure to drink plenty of liquids, especially pure water. Obviously, if God leads you to undertake an absolute fast, you should obey. If so, be certain, without doubt, that God is leading you.

Water-only fasts that last for more than a few days need to be undertaken with a great deal of rest and under medical supervision because of the extreme danger of over-toxification, breakdown of vital body tissues, and loss of electrolytes.

Water and juice fasting or partial fasting may be preferable if you are going to fast for an extended period of time (more than three days). This will provide you with more energy than absolute or water-only fasts and provide the humbling experience of denying your desire for solid food.

Going Beyond Food

During your fast you may feel convicted to refrain from other fleshly desires and things of the world as well. After all, this is what fasting is all about - not satisfying the needs and desires of the flesh, to focus on your relationship with God.

In Paul's letter to the Corinthians, he mentions the practice of abstaining from your marital sexual relations during fasting. *Defraud ye not one the other, except it be with consent for a time, that ye may give yourselves to fasting and prayer; and come together again, that Satan tempt you not for your incontinency.* **1 Corinthians 7:5**

This is not required. It is a decision between you and God, which then you must obviously discuss with your spouse. Other things you may feel you need to refrain from during this time include:

✦ Watching television or movies, playing video games

✦ Reading the newspaper, magazines or other secular reading materials

✦ Listening to secular music

✦ Other various forms of recreation-internet, shopping, talking on phone, etc.

✦ Sleep (instead, pray and worship)

We are all different, and we are all at different levels in our commitment and relationship to God. Whatever it is that God shows you is what you need to be obedient to... and not just because you heard that is what someone else did.

It may be shopping, including in catalogs and on the internet (not for necessities, but for frivolous things), wearing makeup, wearing jewelry, wearing expensive clothes, having your nails done, all these things that are of the world. They have nothing to do with your relationship to God. God doesn't care what we look like on the outside; He cares about the purity of our hearts. If there is something that you think, "*Oh, I couldn't do that,*" the question then becomes, "*Why not?*" We are to let nothing come between us and God. (This is idolatry.)

But seek ye first the kingdom of God, and his righteousness; and all these things shall be added unto you.
Matthew 6:33

Note: The more difficult it is for you to give up these things, the more likely that it is something you need to do. God may want to reveal to you how much power these things have over you (that it has become a stronghold). You need to let God break that. In most cases, after the stronghold is broken, you will have no desire to return to these things! That is when it starts to get exciting. Now you are beginning to recognize strongholds in your life that you were blinded to before!

If you are truly seeking God, but there is an area in your life that is interfering with your relationship with Him, this is the area He is likely to test you on. For example, several times the Bible warns us that personal gain and finances will interfere with our relationship with God.

Then Jesus, beholding him, loved him, and said unto him, One thing thou lackest: go thy way, sell whatsoever thou hast, and give to the poor, and thou shalt have treasure in heaven: and come, take up the cross, and follow me. And he was sad at that saying, and went away grieved: for he had great possessions. And Jesus looked round about, and saith unto his disciples, How hardly shall they that have riches enter into the kingdom of God! And the disciples were astonished at his words. But Jesus answereth again, and saith unto them, Children, how hard is it for them that trust in riches to enter into the kingdom of God! It is easier for a camel to go through the eye of a needle, than for a rich man to enter into the kingdom of God. **Mark 10:21-25**

If God told you to sell everything that you have, give the money to the poor and follow Him, would you? How many people do you know who would be willing to make that sacrifice? *For where your treasure is, there will your heart be also.* **Matthew 6:21**

What do we put before God?

1. Self (personal problems, health problems, circumstances, etc.) - It's not about you!

2. Flesh (we want and crave things such as unhealthy foods, sex, relationships, etc., and have many fleshly desires - which includes our emotions,

179

that can easily over rule what is really best for us - and what God wants for us.)

3. Spouse or personal relationships

4. Work and finances

5. Personal gain, social status, power

6. Family

Anything in your life that becomes more important than God and your relationship with Him becomes a form of idolatry. Don't forget, this is the very first commandment; *Thou shalt have no other gods before me.* **Exodus 20:3**

If we are not seeking Him, if God is not **first** in our lives, if we are not willing to give up everything for him, He will still seek us just as a shepherd will leave the herd to find a lost sheep. **(Matthew 18:11-18)**

The Wilderness

There are three different 40-day fasts mentioned in the Bible. Moses, Elijah and Jesus each went 40 days without food or water. These three fasts also had something of great significance in common. Each of these three individuals was in the wilderness during the fast.

In the wilderness, they were each alone with God. They had no other human distractions. Satan will try to distract us plenty, we don't need to add to it.

Moses: *And he was there with the LORD 40 days and 40 nights; he did neither eat bread, nor drink water. And* he wrote upon the tables the words of the covenant, the ten commandments. **Exodus 34:28**

Elijah: *But he himself went a day's journey into the wilderness...* 1Kings 19:4 *And he arose, and did eat and drink, and went in the strength of that meat 40 days and 40 nights unto Horeb the mount of God.* **1 Kings 19:8**

Jesus: *And Jesus being full of the Holy Ghost returned from Jordan, and was led by the Spirit into the wilderness, Being 40 days tempted of the devil. And in those days he did eat nothing: and when they were ended, he afterward hungered.* **Luke 4:1-3**

When I fast (especially in a prolonged fast) one of my greatest frustrations I feel is the distractions from the world. At this time, when you are sincerely trying to seek God's face, when you are forcing down the desires of the flesh, every day, by not eating, you are professing to God, *"You are more important than food. You are more important than my physical, fleshly, human needs. This much I love you God and I want you first in my life!"*

Experiencing the uprise of the Holy Spirit manifesting within myself, I personally found that my heightened sensitivity to the ick of the world and all the distractions you want to avoid to keep your focus on God, almost becomes unbearable.

Personally, I feel the alone time (with God) required at this time is of the utmost tremendous importance. God will be drawing you to Him and if anything is holding you back or is causing interference, it becomes an inner battle that you do not want to fight. If you can't go forward, in my opinion, you have lost the whole purpose of the fast, which is to experience God! To have God reveal Himself to you!

I feel this is why God gave the three Biblical examples we have, instruction to go to the wilderness, to be alone. Alone with God. No worldly distractions. No people around you cooking, offering you food, creating temptations that need not be present; no one questioning you as to why you are not eating, or if you are losing weight or whatever. People, with good intentions, will tell you that your health is in danger, that only those led by the Holy Spirit should undergo a 40 day fast (as if someone on their own willingness would give up solid food for 40 days) and other things to distract you from what God is calling you to.

I know many people fast (for 40 days even) and otherwise continue life as usual, but I seriously have to wonder how one can really experience all that God has for them in this time if special arrangements are not made for some serious alone time with God. Because I live alone, my only "human" distraction is my dalmatian, KC (because she thinks she's human), so I cannot imagine trying to fast with a house full of people. It is a very intimate time where God wants to speak to you as much as you want to speak to Him and to hear from Him. If there are other people present, going on with their life watching television, listening to music, having friends over socially, etc., how can you hear God?

I strongly encourage you, if at all possible, for a period of time to "go into the wilderness" if God is calling you to fast. If you live alone, tell those you need to that you will not be available for whatever length of time you choose. This may be a weekend, a long weekend, a week, two weeks or however long you can. In this time, turn off the ringer on your phone and let the machine take messages that you (if you desire) can check at your convenience, so not to be interrupted or distracted during crucial times. This is also good discipline demonstrating that no phone call is more important than God. For some people, this may be harder than not eating.

Make any other preparations you need to do such as to stock up on juice and water, etc, so that you will not have to go out. Try to limit your communication with "the world" as much as possible. Do not watch the news, read the newspaper or do any of the other worldly things that you might otherwise do. It is also a good idea (to reduce temptation) to get rid of as much food from the refrigerator as possible. Freeze what you can.

If you do not live alone, at least for a a few days, try to go somewhere (a lake or mountain cabin, find someone who travels and house sit for them, etc.) by yourself, where you will not be interrupted and distracted.

Personally, in my first 40 day fast, it was my intention to do this for three days and I ended up "staying there" for the rest of the fast which was almost two more weeks.

Obviously, not everyone has this luxury because of work or family obligations, but I simply encourage you to do so if you can for part of the fast. The latter part of the fast is preferable, as the further you are into the fast, the more of the Holy Spirit will be present.

If you are married and you both feel that the fast is something you should do together, I think that would be awesome. You could support each other during the rough times (yes, there will be rough times), and it would surely bind that three-strand cord even tighter, but you should also be sure that there is adequate time for each of you to spend individually with God as well.

It is usually easier to fast with someone or with a group of individuals (for any length of time) - such as a prayer partner or prayer team who may not be necessarily physically together. As this is not the focus of this book, I will not be covering this in detail, but it is a very powerful thing to fast in unity with others.

The Significance of 40

The number 40 is used several times in the Bible. It is often used in times of probation, testing, ending in victory or defeat

After Noah built the ark it rained for 40 days and 40 nights (**Genesis 7:4,12**). Forty lashes was often given as a punishment. *Forty stripes he may give him, and not exceed: lest, if he should exceed, and beat him above these with many stripes, then thy brother should seem vile unto thee.* **Deuteronomy 25:3**

The Israelites wandered about the desert for 40 years. Why? *And you shall (earnestly) remember all the way which your Lord your God led you these 40 years in the wilderness, to humble you and to prove you, to know what was in your (mind and) heart, whether you would keep his commandments or not. And HE hum-*

bled you... that HE might make you recognize and per-sonally know that man does not live by bread alone, but man lives by every word that proceeds out of the mouth of the Lord. **Deuteronomy 8:2-3** AMP

Ezekiel was told that a day represented a year, *lie again on thy right side, and thou shalt bear the iniquity of the house of Judah 40 days: I have appointed thee each day for a year.* **Ezekiel 4:6**

God gave the Ninevites 40 days to repent from their wickedness. They proclaimed a fast, repented; God spared them. **Jonah 3:3**

The 40 days Jesus was in the wilderness, He was tempted. Tempted, according to the Greek translation, can also mean "tested" as the Israelites were tested for 40 years. Jesus told Satan, *It is written, Man shall not live by bread alone, but by every word that proceedeth out of the mouth of God.* **Matthew 4:4**

Nutritional Concerns

When fasting longer than three days, you may con-sider juice and water fasts using diluted fruit and veg-etable juices. The natural sugars in juices provide ener-gy, and the taste are motivational to continue your fast.

Whenever possible, it is best to drink fresh juice containing live food enzymes to aid digestion and cleansing in the body. If available, a juicer works great to provide fresh fruit and vegetable juices rich in nutri-tional value and live enzymes.

Also acceptable are juices which contain 100% juice with no sugar or other additives. But remember, unless they are fresh, they contain no enzymes to help detox the body. I suggest that you dilute these juices with water (about 1/2 and 1/2) to help lower the sugar content and glycemic index.

Juice suggestions:

Apple

Carrot

Note: Carrot juice is extremely high in natural sugar so be very careful not to consume high amounts (more than one glass daily). I also suggest diluting carrot juice and your fruit juices and other juices high in natural sugar with water. You can also add some of the pulp back into the juice to help slow down the sugar absorption or another source of fiber such as 1 tablespoon of freshly ground flax seeds.

Grape - concord or white

Cucumber

Celery

Cabbage

Beet

Kale

Spinach

Watermelon (with seeds removed), raspberries and other similar fruits can be placed in the blender and pureed. Add other juice or water to the desired consistency.

Green juice-blend such as celery, romaine lettuce, and carrots in equal proportions.

"Green drinks" containing chlorella, wheat grass, barley green or spirulina are excellent de-toxifiers.

There are many excellent fruit varieties available frozen as well which are great as long as they are 100% fruit juice (no added sweeteners!).

Make a warm vegetable broth: Gently boil sliced potatoes, carrots, celery, onion, garlic, cabbage, broccoli, etc., in water. Do not add salt. After about a half-hour, drain off the water and drink. Any extra will keep in the fridge for several days.

Hot apple cider (diluted with water) and hot herbal tea are also acceptable.

Orange and tomato juice are not recommended in large amounts because their acidic content may cause an upset stomach in some, although processed low-acid orange juice is now available for purchase in most grocery stores. These juices also are better tolerated if diluted with equal portions of water.

I like to warm up tomato juice (diluted with water) and add some cayenne pepper to stimulate the circulation as I tend to feel very cold when I fast.

Before You Begin

As you begin your fast, family and friends may urge you to protect your health, and you should. But if done properly, fasting will not only prove to be a spiritual, but a physical blessing as well.

If you have any health concerns, consult your doctor before you begin your fast. But, be aware that many doctors have not been trained in this area and, therefore, their understanding is limited. You may have a physical problem that would make fasting unwise or dangerous. Also, if you are taking any type of medication, make sure you talk to your doctor before changing your regime. Prudence, wisdom and caution are in order.

In spite of the absolute safety and benefits of fasting, there are certain persons who should not fast on juice and water alone, unless you know for sure that God has directed you to do exactly so. Partial fasting should be acceptable for most (even diabetics and children). For example:

✦ Individuals who are physically too thin or emaciated.

✦ Individuals who are prone to anorexia, bulimia, or other behavioral disorders. (Unless you are fasting specifically to break free from these bondages.)

✦ Individuals who suffer weakness or anemia or other nutritional deficiencies.

✦ Individuals who suffer serious chronic problems with kidneys, liver, lungs, heart or other organs.

✦ Individuals who take insulin for diabetes, or suffer any other blood sugar problem such as hypoglycemia.

✦ Women who are nursing, pregnant or trying to get pregnant.

Before you begin your fast, decide (and even write it down) what your intentions are:

✦ Is there a specific purpose for your fast? (Your fast may be simply in obedience to what God has called you to do or you may be seeking deliverance from a specific problem, etc.)

✦ How long will you fast?

✦ What do you intend to fast from (solid food, meat, sugar, sweets, coffee, chocolate, processed food)?

✦ What (foods or drink) will you allow?

✦ Do you have any specific spiritual goals or questions you want answered?

Keep in mind that when Jesus was asked a question by His disciples or the Pharisees, He often did not answer their question in the way that they expected, while He did, none-the-less, answer their question. You may have already seen in your own life, that this is often how God works as well. So, as you may have specific questions in mind that you would like answers for, God may have some very different things in mind that He wants to show you. He may indeed answer your questions... but He may not do so in the way you expected, so you may not recognize it as such right away.

If you are on a water and juice fast, do not consume milk or other dairy products because they are food and therefore a violation of the fast. Products containing protein or fat, such as milk, yogurt, kefir, rice or soy-based drinks, should also be avoided. These products will restart digestion and will stir up hunger.

Caffeinated beverages such as coffee, black tea, and pop should be avoided. Caffeine is a stimulant; it has a more powerful effect on your nervous system when you abstain from food. They are highly acidic and are also diuretics which further depletes your body of important nutrients faster than normal.

Do not chew gum as it stimulates the digestive system and could cause hunger.

Preparing for a Short-term Fast

If you plan on fasting for a short period of time (3-10 days) you should find the following suggestions helpful:

✦ A day or two before your fast is to begin, start eating smaller meals. Resist the urge to have that "last big meal" before the fast as this will only create more hunger in the first few days of the fast. Cutting down on your food intake signals your mind, stomach, and appetite that less food is acceptable.

✦ Consider eating only raw foods for a day or two days before starting.

✦ Before your fast, wean yourself off of caffeine and sugar products to ease your initial hunger or discomfort at the early stages of your fast.

Preparing for a Long-term Fast

If you are considering a prolonged fast (longer than 3 days) of juice and water, it is wise to prepare your body prior to your start date. Here are some suggestions in addition to those above for a short-term fast.

✦ Consider eating a vegetable diet (mostly raw) for a week or so before starting. Slowly decrease the total volume of food you consume. In other words, for several days before you start, eat light.

✦ About 3 days (or longer if you wish) before your fast, you will want to begin cleansing your colon. Do this by adding 1-2 heaping table-spoons of freshly ground flax (rich in fiber) to a tall glass of juice or smoothie in the morning, and in a glass of juice again in the evening. If your bowels do not move by the second day, you are probably not drinking enough water. You can also increase your flax-juice to three times a day if needed. If desired, continue the flax-juice 1 time a day for several days into your fast to continue cleansing the bowels. (Keep in mind flax seeds are a whole food providing calories and nutrients, so you must consider if this "food" belongs in your fast.)

An alternative to flax is inulin, another great fiber to add to water, tea or juice. Inulin can be used before and perhaps even throughout your entire fast. This is a soluble fiber which completely disolves in your liquid. It has very few calories, about 8 per teaspoon. You may be very surprized at how much waste you continue to move out of your body after you begin your fast. This is a good thing as the fast is giving your body a chance to completely get cleaned out!

Comments on Laxatives and Colon Cleansing

Laxatives (including natural herbs such as cascara sagrada and senna), colonics and enemas are too harsh and disrupt the body's balance. They, like a drug, force the body to do something, rather than naturally encourage it to perform it's normal function (as the fiber in the flax will do). I also prefer the ground flax (a whole food) over a fiber isolate such as psyllium husks. If we had enough fiber in our diet, we would never need to take laxatives or need "colon cleansing."

The recommended daily intake of fiber is 25-30 grams, but the average American intake is only 11 grams! No wonder we have epidemics of weight problems, constipation and colon cancer!

I do not recommend laxatives (including harsh laxative herbs), colonics and enemas because:

1. They do not just flush waste out of the colon, they strip it of the natural bacteria (flora) that need to be present to maintain good intestinal health.

2. They are very easy to overuse, abuse and are highly addictive as the bowels quickly (in only a few days of use) lose their ability to move without stimulation. Herbs such as senna, cascara sagrada, buckthorn and others are only meant for brief and rare use in extreme conditions. All colon cleansers are meant to provide only temporary symptomatic relief. They do so by irritating the lining of the colon. As a result, the bowels do not move in the natural way they are intended to after you eat a meal. Instead, the entire intestinal tract goes into spasms (known as griping, which can be very painful) and the entire bowel is eventually evacuated, usually within 24 hours.

3. This also prevents nutrients and minerals from being absorbed properly, creating electrolyte mineral deficiencies (especially of potassium), and disturbances in acid-base (pH) balance. (Baker)

There are actual deaths associated with long-term daily use of these natural herbal laxatives. Toxicologists report that these herbs can cause an electrolyte imbalance so serious it can lead to muscle and heart ailments, including arrhythmia and heart failure. Chronic use of laxatives is also associated with increased risk of colon cancer, renal failure and Calcareous. (Copeland, Wu)

Calcareous are abnormal stones formed by mineral salts clumped together caused by improper pH and mineral imbalances. These stones can occur in any tissue in the body, common places include the kidneys, gallbladder, urinary tract and joints.

Our Health in Fasting...Using WISDOM!

When we stop eating in a fast, a great deal of energy (otherwise needed to digest food) becomes available for the body to take care of it's natural responsibility to cleanse and detoxify itself. The digestive process of breaking down of the food we do eat, requires a tremendous amount of energy. (notice how tired you will feel after eating a big meal). A diet high in cooked and processed foods adds to the burden as all of our own pancreatic enzymes are needed to help break down the food. Raw foods eaten contain the natural enzymes God placed there to aid in our digestion of them. Enzymes are destroyed in cooking and processing of food.

In addition to helping us break down food, our pancreatic enzymes also cleanse and detoxify the body. During a fast as they are not needed for digestion, these enzymes then can go do this work elsewhere in the body. (This is also why it is important to eat a diet high in raw foods - it relieves the burden of pancreatic enzyme to do these other things. This process of detoxification of the body releases toxins from our cells and tissues creating an acidic environment in our body. Because of this, it is very important to not compound the problem by consuming acid-forming juices and beverages. On page 210 you can see that coffee, black tea and sweetened fruit juice are highly acidic and therefore should be AVOIDED!

Our blood is so important that God designed the body (fearfully and wonderfully) to maintain homeostasis (balance). If the body fluids become acidic, to neutralize the acidity in the blood, the body will take alkalizing agents to buffer it. The body does this with minerals. (This is why milk, Milk of Magnesia™ and Tums™ are antidotes for hyperacidity in the stomach.) If we do not have adequate minerals in the digestive system to use for this purpose, the body will take them from our bones.

Unfortunately, I have seen the negative physical effects of long-term (improper) fasting. It was a painful thing to me for God to show me mighty men and women of God, who I greatly respect, who had been faithfully serving Him through fasting, who were now suffering the physical consequences with altered metabolism and spinal degeneration and other health problems. For years as I waited for God to give me the release to publish this book, I cried out to God, "What is it you are trying to show me? What is missing? What do you want me to do with this book?"

In February of 2003 when I was preparing to teach on fasting at IHOP in Kansas City, MO, God clearly spoke to me about His concerns with His people fasting today. He said,

"Toxic. My people are toxic. The land is toxic. The soil and water does not provide the minerals it did even 100 years ago. Coral calcium and other supplements can provide the minerals my

people need during fasting that are no longer pro-
vided in the water. The world will try to manipu-
late you, the enemy wants to destroy you. Use
wisdom."

I finally realized what He is trying to tell me. Years ago our drinking water was a major source of minerals and trace minerals. But today, we rarely drink pure natural water from wells or springs. City water is processed and then treated with chemicals. Distilled water is pure, but all the minerals have been removed along with the contaminants. Those minerals that water once provided are of crucial importance to our health in fasting. We clearly need to be getting these minerals into the body to prevent acidosis and the health problems that result. Water is a diuretic, so if we are drinking water without minerals, we are addition-ally flushing valuable needed minerals out of the body!

I have never been convicted to stop taking my sup-plements when I fast. While I was curious as to why, now I clearly understand that God was protecting my health, knowing I was not going to get those minerals any other way.

If the land is toxic, that means that the food grown in that soil also does not contain the nutrients that these foods once did. Our foods can only be as healthy as the soil it is grown in. So even juicing fresh, organic fruits and vegetables may not be adequate to provide us what we need.

Coral Calcium Minerals

One mighty man of God with a tremendous healing ministry, Cal Pierce, Director of the Healing Rooms in Spokane, WA, was specifically instructed by God to take coral calcium minerals during a 40-day fast. He said that he had more energy than ever before during such a fast and also reported that he did not as quickly regain the weight he had lost during the fast when he stopped fasting. This is of great significance to him.

Coral calcium minerals are available as a food supplement made from ocean coral that provides calcium, magnesium, sulfur, silicon and 70+ other minerals and in similar proportion to the level they are found in the blood. Coral calcium minerals has a much better absorption rate than many other calcium supplements because of the way it is enzymatically formed by the sea creatures that live there. The same minerals found in coral are the same minerals found in sea water and the dust of the earth... which we are made of! **(Genesis 2:7)**

Medical science does not give much significance to over 75% of the different minerals in the body, mostly because they are in trace amounts and/or we don't know what function they play in our health. If God put them in our body, no matter how minute in quantity, just because we don't know WHY, does not make them any less important!

So... if our food and water are not providing these minerals, and if we are using them up because our systems are acidic and toxic, the potential for health problems should be of no surprise.

We need to make sure we have a reliable source of

minerals during fasting. We need to avoid acid-forming substances (see pages 192-193), **especially** during fasting, to ward off future health problems. God is NOT telling us NOT to fast, He is telling us to USE WISDOM when fasting. He is reminding us that His people perish for lack of knowledge.

Personally, I have found that when I fast I may need to almost double my intake of coral minerals during fasting to keep my body's pH healthy, which is slightly alkaline (7.4). Fasting puts your body into "detox" mode which quickly creates an acidic environment. When fasting, I strongly suggest you frequently check your pH (at least once per day) to ensure your body is not getting too acidic. PH test strips are available at many drug stores and through the internet.

If one brand of coral calcium minerals does not work for you, try another. Unfortunately, not all manufacturing and marketing companies have integrity. There are also other multi-mineral sources that are available and beneficial, other than coral calcium that can be used.

Cucumbers!

In one fast I was on, God told me I could eat cucumbers! (I was really happy about this because my parents had just given me a bunch of cucumbers from their garden!) You can see that cucumbers are one of the most alkaline foods we can eat. It ranks right up there with wheat grass!!

Wheat grass . . . . +34
Cucumbers (fresh) . . . . +31
Soy sprouts . . . . +30

Alfalfa grass .... +29
Barley grass .... +28
Radishes (red) .... +28

In your fasting, don't be so religious! Ask God what He wants you to do, how He wants you to fast. He knows what your body needs! Ask Him for wisdom, He will give it to you.

Fasting, Minerals and Metabolism

Metabolism is the rate at which the body burns calories for energy. It is largely regulated by hormones produced by the thyroid and adrenal glands.

There are four main minerals which regulate and in turn are regulated by the activity of the adrenal and thyroid glands. These metabolic regulators are calcium (Ca), magnesium (Mg), sodium (Na), and potassium (K). All four of these minerals need to be at normal levels for the thyroid and adrenal glands to supply maximum amounts of energy. A minor fluctuation in one of these minerals can cause either one or both of these glands to become either under-active or over-active.

Other important minerals which play a significant role in the optimal functioning of the thyroid are iodine and selenium. (Zimmermann, Kohrle) Modern day agricultural practices have already greatly depleted our soil of these important minerals in many parts of the world. Studies show that deficiencies of these minerals cause numerous health problems, including hypothyroidism (low thyroid functioning). (Bertoli) Hypothyroidism is associated with weight gain and obesity.

Another very important trace mineral commonly deficient in our modern processed diets of today is chromium. Chromium is needed for insulin to bring glucose into our cells for burning as fuel. Without adequate amount, the glucose cannot enter the cells (making them insulin resistant) and the glucose is stored instead. Therefore, chromium is crucially important for energy production, blood sugar metabolism and fat burning.

Because of the increased risk of mineral loss during fasting due to increased acidosis, compounded with the natural slow down in the metabolic rate due to not eating, the risk of rapid weight gain after a fast has ended is a serious risk for which precautions should be taken. The best ways to do this is to:

1. **Slowly** (over several days) **increase your caloric intake after a fast.** Your stomach will shrink, so this may not be difficult for the first day, but once you start eating, your hunger will quickly be returned and it will be returned in great magnitude. If you do not make a serious conscientious effort to control your eating you may be eating everything in sight. Because your metabolism will be greatly slowed down, your body will be storing most of these new calories, instead of burning them.

While weight loss is not your concern (focus) when fasting for the Lord, you may lose 10, 20, 30 or more pounds in a 40 day juice/water fast. BUT, if you are not careful, you may gain it all back in less than one week, and then gain some extra, due to your depressed metabolic rate. This is extremely stressful to the body and very unhealthy! The older you are, and the less healthy the state of your glands, especially the thyroid, the longer it will take for your body to adjust after a fast, so you need to be very careful to prevent unwanted rapid weight gain.

2. Make sure you are getting an adequate supply of minerals throughout your fast to not further suppress the activity of your glands and metabolic activity of the body. When your fast is completed, your thyroid cannot return to it's proper level of metabolic functioning if it does not have the proper minerals to do so. The same applies to all other organs and glands in the body that have been affected by the fast.

This can easily be done through a supplement like coral calcium (which contains about 74 different minerals which are all found in the body) as I have mentioned earlier. Every single one of these minerals is important in it's function in the body. Just because medical science has not yet discovered WHAT function it plays in the body, does not lesson it's importance. God would not have put all those minerals in our body for no reason! EACH one, no matter how small an amount is needed, IS very important for our health.

Frequent fasting can cause serious mineral imbalances and serious health problems. I have seen too many people compromise their health while they believed they were being obedient to the Lord to fast. I sincerely believe this is one of the primary reasons I have been directed to write this book.

3. Suggested foods to eat and not to eat imediately following a prolonged fast (10 days or more):

I have had to learn these things the hard way of course, so here is my advise:

<u>**Acceptable foods to eat in the first few days following a long fast:**</u>
1. **Steamed vegetables** - especially green ones
2. **Fresh fruit**
3. **Yogurt, kifer** or other probiotic-containing dairy products

<u>**After a few more days you can add:**</u>
1. **Poached or softboiled eggs**
2. **Fish**
3. **Whole grain bread**
4. **Whole grains like steel-cut oats, barley, wild rice, etc.**
5. **Almonds**
6. **Cheese**

<u>**Avoid for several days:**</u>
1. **Salads and other raw vegetables**
2. **Meat** (especially red meat)
3. **Other nuts and seeds** (almonds are the only alkaline nuts, all others are acidic.)
4. **Beans** (if they are hard for you to digest - it varies person to person, I don't have a problem with them, but some people do, so I am including it)

These foods are harder to digest and may cause diarrhea or stomach upset.

Physical Effects... What to Expect

In a nutshell, I would have to say that fasting is a physically, emotionally, and spiritually grueling experience. But, most people (who are truly fasting to God) will tell you that it is, indeed, worth every minute.

In this time of discipline, self-sacrifice and reflection, do not be surprised if you experience mental (emotional) and physical discomforts. When you talk to different people about the physical effects of fasting, you get many different comments as everyone responds in different ways. Many things vary according to the amount of experience the faster has, the type of diet the faster normally has, one's individual physical body size, etc. Here are some general things:

✦ As you stop eating, during days two through four, your metabolism will start slowing down in accordance with how many calories you are consuming through juice. In this process and for the rest of the fast, you are likely to feel cold. It is likely that you will need or want to put on an extra layer of clothes to maintain comfort. The less body fat you have the more cold you are likely to feel. If you feel cold, try drinking hot herbal tea, broth, or going for a walk to stimulate blood flow.

A word of advice of what NOT to do if you feel cold: Cayenne pepper is commonly recommended for people with poor circulation who tend to feel cold a lot. I often supplement cayenne pepper capsules in the winter months to encourage optimal circulation. When you are fasting, however, this is NOT a good idea. I tried it one time when I was fasting in the winter months with subzero temperatures outside and found I became so nauseous I ended up throwing up - which upset my electrolytes and ended up not feeling well for a couple of days. If you want to add a sprinkle of cayenne pepper to a vegetable broth, this should be alright, but don't overdo it like I did by taking a whole capsules! It's powerful stuff.

✦ You are likely to have less energy and require more sleep, especially in the beginning of your fast as your body is adjusting. You may need to take short naps.

✦ You may need to limit your physical activity. Exercise only moderately and rest as much as your schedule permits (especially for extended fasts).

✦ Walking at a moderate pace will help stimulate blood flow, making you feel rejuvenated. Those on a water-only fast should not exercise.

✦ Hunger: The degree of hunger experienced from person to person varies greatly. For many people on a prolonged fast, the most hunger is experienced in the first few days. However, physical activity, the smell of food, being around food and other things can stimulate hunger. If you feel hungry, increase your water intake.

✦ Also expect to go the the bathroom more often because you should be drinking lots of water!

The following is a list of additional possible effects, possible causes and solutions:

✦ **Lower back pain:** This may indicate that you are dehydrated. Drink more water!

✦ **Bad breath, heightened body odor, feeling of heaviness or achiness in muscles,** and **acne breakouts** may result as cells are releasing toxins. Drink more water. Adding MSM (organic source of sulfur) to your water can help speed up the detoxification process. Add about 1 teaspoon to 12 oz. of water three times daily.

Alfalfa, chlorella and barley green are rich in chlorophyll, a natural body deodorizer, and can help control bad breath and gently cleanse the system. Take two to four 500 mg. tablets at a time two to three times daily. (Note: An empty stomach may be sensitive to alfalfa, so you may need to take it with juice.)

✦ **A white or yellow-coated tongue** may be a part of the body's pattern of throwing off toxins. Drink more water and consider adding MSM. A yellow color indicates a higher level of acidity. This may be from excess sugar, refined foods, coffee. etc, in your diet. You may want to consider altering your diet after the fast is over (to a healthier one).

✦ **Changes in elimination** (constipation or diarrhea), can be aided by drinking more water. Mix two tablespoons of freshly ground flax seed mixed with 8 oz. of juice two to three times per day to help in elimination and cleansing and also to reduce hunger pangs.

✦ **Light-headedness** may result from quickly standing up or changing positions. Try to move more slowly and cautiously. Also could indicate blood pressure changes. Check your urine pH for mineral status.

✦ **Headaches** or **stomachaches** may be a result of salt, sugar, or caffeine withdrawal. Peppermint herbal tea can be helpful for stomach upset. Also try to drink more water. Eliminating those items from your diet prior to fasting is the best way to avoid these.

✦ **Nausea** accompanied by weakness towards the end of a prolonged fast may be a warning sign that you are severely nutrient/energy depleted and you may want to make a juice drink, adding a small amount (one teaspoon) of freshly ground flax seed and whey protein powder (one teaspoon). A greens drink from chlorella, spirulina or wheat grass would also be beneficial. Just be sure to sip it slowly.

Nausea may also result in some individuals taking nutritional supplements on an empty stomach. Switch to liquid supplements if possible.

Nausea may also be an indication of excess stomach acidity. This can be aided by increasing vegetable juices such as from greens, cucumber, beet, celery, etc.

✦ Changes in **sleeping and dreaming** patterns could be sugar or caffeine withdrawal symptoms. Try drinking more water. Valerian or chamomile tea in the evening may be helpful for disturbed sleep.

If you are experiencing many detox symptoms, you may want to also consider supplementing silymarin (Milk thistle extract) or alpha lipoic acid to help support, protect and enhance the cleansing of the liver.

✦ **Cravings:** Often (not always) cravings for specific foods are caused by a certain nutritional deficiency and this creates an overwhelming desire of the body for that nutrient. Often it is a mineral. (These cravings also apply for times other than when fasting.) If more than one nutrient deficiency is listed as a possible cause, to help you determine which one, look at the foods which are high in that specific mineral and consider if this is also a food you are craving.

Sugar cravings: This could be the result of a chromium deficiency. Juices which are high in the trace mineral chromium are recommended: These include apple, green pepper, spinach, carrot and potato. You could also try adding brewer's yeast to your juice. You could also be addicted to sugar, for which chromium should still be helpful.

Chocolate cravings: Could be due to lack of copper or magnesium. Juices high in copper include: apple, carrot, garlic, ginger root and coconut. Juices high in magnesium include: beet greens, spinach, parsley, garlic, carrot and celery.

Salt cravings: While it may be a sodium deficiency (NOT sodium chloride or table salt), it is much more likely to be a lack of potassium. Juices which are high in potassium include parsley, garlic, spinach and carrot. It could also be from stress to the adrenal glands. Juices recommended include: Ginger, parsley, potato, garlic, carrot, green pepper, kale, cauliflower, beet greens. To help maintain mineral balances on a daily basis use sea salt instead of regular table salt.

Peanut butter or nut cravings: Increase minerals, especially copper. Juices high in copper include: apple, carrot, garlic, ginger root, and coconut. Also rich in copper: oysters, nuts, split peas, liver, buckwheat.

Sour cravings: Could be acetic acid deficiency. Increase lemon and lime juice. Chlorophyll (found in deep green foods) is also helpful.

If you experience severe pain or swelling, you should stop your fast.

Note: The use of nutritional supplements during your fasting is between you and God. If you feel convicted that it is not something God is directing you to do, then you need to be obedient to that. I have felt (with God's approval) that I needed to continue my supplements (especially high amounts of coral calcium) during fasting. I also sometimes add chlorella, barley green or wheat grass to my juice to help maintain proper pH in the body and provide a wide variety of trace nutrients. Chlorella, barley green and wheat grass are also rich in chlorophyll, an excellent natural detoxifier. For more information on this, see my book, *Chlorella: The Ultimate Green Food.*

Emotional/Mental Effects... What to Expect

Especially in a prolonged fast of self-denial of the pleasure of eating delicious food, it is likely that you will experience times of impatience, irritability, fear, anxiety, frustration, depression, grief, utter devastation and humility. However, there will also be times that you will experience complete joy, freedom, elation, as you float in the glory clouds of heaven's peace and closeness to God.

Even through the negative feelings and even if you feel you have failed, you will note an underlying sense of peace of knowing that this is what God has called you to do.

An increased spiritual awareness should occur during your fast as you renew your closeness with God Not everyone will have a "mountaintop experience" every time they fast. Fasting can be physically, emotionally and spiritually grueling, but you need to remember that your fast is not about what you are going to get out of it, but it is an act of worship to God. When your motives are right, God will honor your seeking heart and bless your time with Him.

During your fast, you will surely have your struggles, discomforts, spiritual victories and failures. As you are stripped down to the bare bones of complete reliance upon God and humility and weakness, there will be times where the flesh seems to rise up out of nowhere as if your body is crying out, *"Hello? I'm human, I can't do this!"*

In the morning you may feel great, but by evening you may be irritable, frustrated and wrestling with the flesh, sorely tempted to raid the refrigerator and counting how many more days are left in your fast. This is especially true in the beginning of a fast and if you are new at fasting.

Fight temptations with prayer. Take extra time to spend with God. Step outside for fresh air and a moderate walk. Pray and seek God's comfort as you walk. Sing songs of praise and worship. And in the process always keep on sipping water or diluted juice frequently during your waking hours.

While some people like rigid schedules, I suggest avoiding making a time table of when you are going to drink your juice. If you do try to make a schedule, you may find yourself clock-watching, instead of letting the Spirit lead you in all you do at this time.

People have described their fasting schedule of carrot juice for breakfast and apple juice for lunch and etc., and I thought, "this is a fast; there is no such thing as breakfast, lunch and dinner!"

As you enter this time of heightened spiritual devotion, Satan will do everything he can to pull you away from your prayer and Bible study time. When you feel the enemy trying to discourage you, immediately pray and ask God to strengthen you in the face of difficulties and temptations.

The enemy makes you a target because he knows that fasting is the most powerful of all Christian disciplines and that God may have something very special to show you as you wait upon Him and seek His face. Satan does not want you to grow in your faith, and will do anything from making you hungry and grumpy to bringing up trouble in your family or at work to stop you. Make prayer your shield against such attacks.

Excuses

"I am too weak to fast"

We all are too weak (in our own strength) to fast on our own. This is part of the humbling process that God calls us to. This is why we need to spend time with God, asking Him for His strength, for His grace.

God told Paul, *My grace is sufficient for thee: for **my strength** is made perfect in (your) weakness. Most gladly therefore will I rather glory in my infirmities, that the power of Christ may rest upon me.* Paul wrote, *Therefore, I take pleasure in infirmities, in reproaches, in necessities, in persecutions, in distresses for Christ's sake: for when I am weak, then am I strong.* **2 Corinthians 12:9-10**

Just thinking about fasting can make me hungry. We need to be in control of our minds and our flesh! Learning to discipline our flesh (and our thoughts) is also an important part of fasting whether it is a total fast or you are just fasting from sugar or coffee. Once we commit to a fast it is very important we stick to it.

"I can't fast, I'm diabetic, I'm hypoglycemic or I get sick if I don't eat"

If you have been reading, you should have realized by now that there are many, many different ways we can fast. We can all find things to fast from.

And if you fail...

What if I mess up? What if I forget or what if I just eat something?

Sometimes we are harder on ourselves than God is. If you eat something that is contrary to your fast, simply repent, ask for forgiveness and go on. There is no reason to abandon the entire fast. This is no reason to "start over" on day one, for example, if you are halfway through a two week fast. This is not the kind of God I serve. God knows how weak we are. He knows our heart. He knows. Talk to Him. Repent and ask Him how He feels about it. When I fail, He usually tells me something like, "I know" or "my strength is made perfect in your weakness."

One time I was fasting (probably 3 days) and I had been outdoors working, which, of course, stirs up our metabolism. I was having a great time praying and singing, enjoying the weather, etc. When I finally finished my task, I was totally exhausted, my whole body ached and I was VERY hungry! I came in the house, went right to the fridge and took out a muffin and started eating it. I only had about two bites left before I realized what I was doing! I gave the rest to KC (my dalmatian), and whined, "Oh God, I was so hungry!" He just said, "I know." He really does. He knows how weak we are. He understands.

For we are glad, when we are weak, and ye are strong: and this also we wish, even your perfection.
2 Corinthians 13:9

Grace

Yes, there will be times that you feel you just don't have the grace to fast. Remember, the bigger the battle you are fighting... the bigger the battle your fast is going to be... BUT, the bigger the VICTORY will be as well!

Some people have great grace for fasting, meaning it is not difficult at all for them to fast for prolonged periods, while other people struggle to get through one day. In seasons I have found tremendous grace to fast, and other times, found it to be extremely challenging. There are times when God will give us the grace, and there are other times, He wants us to be learning discipline. There are other times, where God does not want us to be fasting, but desires that we come into a period of feasting where He wants to love on us and nourish us. We need to be in tune to the Spirit and to what God desires of you at any given time.

Abundance of grace provides the ongoing spiritual resources that are necessary for the development of a godly, victorious walk for the glory of God in the midst of humanity here on earth.

But may the God of all grace, who called us to His eternal glory by Christ Jesus . . . perfect, establish, strengthen, and settle you. **1 Peter 5:10**

Through grace, all those who are called may receive the promise of the eternal inheritance. Meanwhile, until Christ returns for us, He wants to develop our lives spiritually and our relationship with Him during our time here on earth.

God desires to perfect our lives. He calls us to be holy.... through the process of sanctification. God completes what is missing and equips us for His service. The purpose of the anointing is not for us, and for our own glory, it is for **His Glory**! He anoints us to do the work which we could not otherwise accomplish without it (or Him)!

He that has clean hands, and a pure heart; who has not lifted up his soul into vanity (pride), *nor sworn deceitfully. He shall receive the blessing of the Lord, and righteousness from the God of his salvation.* **Psalms 24: 4-5**

Now may the God of peace . . . make you complete in every good work to do His will . . . And He Himself gave some to be apostles, some prophets, some evangelists, and some pastors and teachers, for the equipping of the saints for the work of ministry. **Hebrews 13:20-21** and **Ephesians 4:12**. God's work is done on earth through His servants. It is important that we, as representatives of Him, in a manner pleasing to Him, continue the work that Jesus began when He was here. God makes it clear that there is no room for lukewarm Christians in this mission. It is only through God's grace we can accomplish this.

Finally, God wants us to be ready... to be grounded in His ways... through His word, by our obedience, service, humility, holiness, and most of all, love.

CONCLUSION

If you feel there are areas of this book where I am being harsh, it is because God is calling His children to a higher standard. He is not tolerating mixture – which He calls lukewarm. I have seen (what I believe to be) His judgement fall on those who have failed to step up (to what He's calling them to do) and it's not pretty. He says, "*I will spew thee out of my mouth.*" Please hear me, this is serious. "*Be holy for I am holy*" is not just a suggestion on how to please God and look good in the church. Not at all... He is saying that anything less (than holiness) will be spewed!

God Wants You Well, the title of my first book for God, is largely about physical healing and our responsibility to take care of the body as a temple of the Holy Spirit. I talk about how God healed me (interestingly, *after* I started writing the book), of my lifelong struggle with asthma and how He freed me from the reliance of pharmaceuticals. The healing actually occurred during a time of great personal brokenness.

This book is also about healing; not so much about physical healing, but emotional healing. God wants to heal us of the woundings we carry deep within our soul, but it is something that we must LET Him do. He cannot heal us if we have our walls up, shutting Him out. We cannot have the kind of relationship that God desires of us, as long as we keep our walls up.

Unhealed wounds are the major wall builders which interfere with our communion and relationship with God. These often stem from as far back as our conception and birth, are what causes us to start building this protective shield against further pain. Depending on how long ago these things occurred, there may be layer upon layer upon layer of walls; solid brick, cemented together and stacked high.

These wounds and walls also interfere with our relationships with others on earth and this is another important reason that God wants us to tear them down.

God is calling us to Him. He wants 100% of us. He wants to tear down those walls. We must not allow stagnancy. We must continue to grow in our relationship with Him. We must press in. We must fast, humble ourselves, seek His face and repent. In the brokenness of a fast, God is finally able to start tearing the walls down so the Holy Spirit can start working on us.

Paul wrote: *I press toward the mark for the prize of the high calling of God in Christ Jesus.* **Philippians 3:14**

The only thing that can stand between you and your relationship with God and your walk **in the power of God** is you. God wants to empower you to holiness and to do His kingdom work. **(Hebrews 12:28)**

Press!

Author's Final Notes:

It has been several years since I actually wrote the bulk of this manuscript (during a 40-day fast). Since then God has refined and made important additions for the full revelation of the purpose of this book.

It may be difficult to understand this book without a full revelation of the significance that Christ is soon coming for His bride (the church)... and the bride, in her current state, is not ready. The bride needs to be pure and holy, sanctified in every area of her life for His purpose.

When God is trying to get his message out to the people, He will often deliver it to several of His prophets around the nations. I was blessed to see in July 2003, Rick Joyner posted the following on the Elijah list (a prophetic announcement email posting),

> "Much of the church presently lives in a state which ranges from luke-warmness to a deep spiritual slumber. As the Lord warned in Revelation 3:16, luke-warmness is the worst state a Christian could ever fall into. Many, who are at least to some degree awake, do not know what time it is. The Lord is going to graciously sound an alarm that will wake us up, and declare the time to us as well."

I pray for each reader that you will receive an impartation of the truth, a revelation of the lukewarm areas of your life and of the significance of Christ's coming for His holy bride. His peace and Love I give to you! Beth

BIBLIOGRAPHY

Baker EH, Sandle GI. Complications of laxative abuse. Annu Rev Med 1996;47:127-34.

Bertoli A, Fusco A, Andreoli A, Magnani A, Tulli A, Lauro D, De Lorenzo A.; Effect of subclinical hypothyroidism and obesity on whole-body and regional bone mineral content. Horm Res 2002;57(3-4):79-84.

Ciola, Greg, GMO's; The Food Apocalypse, Crusador Enterprises, Orlando, FL.

Copeland PM.; Renal failure associated with laxative abuse. Eating Disorder Program, Salem Hospital, MA Psychother Psychosom 1994;62(3-4):200-2.

Kohrle J.; The trace element selenium and the thyroid gland. Biochimie 1999 May;81(5):527-33.

Ley, B.; Calcium: The Facts, Fossilized Coral, BL Publications, Detroit Lakes, MN, 2001.

Ley, Chlorella, The Ultimate Green Food, BL Publications, Detroit Lakes, MN, 2003.

Wu WJ, Huang CH, Chiang CP, Huang CN, Wang CN. Urolithiasis related to laxative abuse. Department of Urology, Kaohsiung Medical College, Taiwan, R.O.C. J Formos Med Assoc 1993 Nov;92(11):1004-6.

Zimmermann MB, Kohrle J.; The impact of iron and selenium deficiencies on iodine and thyroid metabolism: biochemistry and relevance to public health. Thyroid 2002 Oct;12(10):867-78.

ABOUT THE AUTHOR

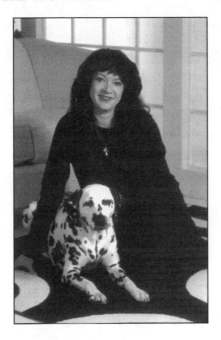

Beth M. Ley, Ph.D., has been a science writer specializing in health and nutrition since 1988 and has written many health-related books, including the best sellers, ***DHEA: Unlocking the Secrets to the Fountain of Youth*** and ***MSM: On Our Way Back to Health With Sulfur.*** She graduated in Scientific and Technical Writing from North Dakota State University in 1987 (combination of Zoology and Journalism). She also has her masters (1997) and doctoral degrees (1999) in Nutrition from Clayton University.

Dr. Beth is dedicated to God and to spreading the health message. Her vision is to help prepare the bride. (Isa. 62:10-12.) In addition to writing, she does nutrition counseling and speaks on Biblical nutrition nationwide.

Memberships: American Nutraceutical Association, New York Academy of Sciences, Resurrection International Apostolic Network (RAIN). Gospel Crusade.

Order these great books from NHL Ministries!

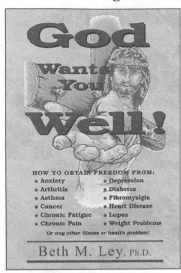

240 pages, $14.95

ISBN: 1-890766-19-4

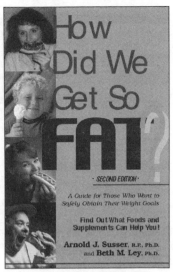

110 pages, $8.95

ISBN: 0-9642703-0-7

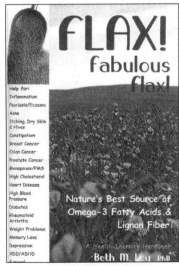

48 pages, $4.95

ISBN: 0-890766-24-0

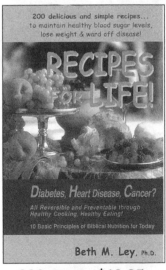

200 pages, $19.95
Spiral Bound Cookbook!
ISBN: 0-890766-29-1

Orders call toll free: 1-877-BOOKS11
Or visit: www.blpublications.com

More great books from NHL Ministries!

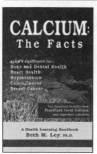
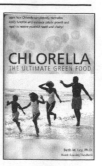
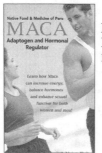
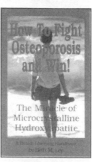
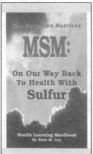
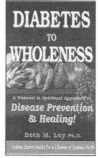
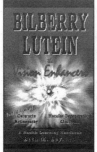
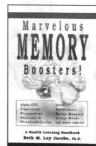

T O   P L A C E   A N   O R D E R :

Aspirin Alternatives: The Top Natural Pain-Relieving Analgesics
____ (Lombardi) $8.95

____ **Bilberry & Lutein: The Vision Enhancers!** (Ley) $4.95

____ **Calcium: The Facts, Fossilized Coral** (Ley) $4.95

____ **Castor Oil: Its Healing Properties** (Ley) $3.95

____ **Dr. John Willard on Catalyst Altered Water** (Ley) $3.95

____ **Chlorella: Ultimate Green Food (Ley)** $4.95

____ **CoQ10: All-Around Nutrient for All-Around Health** (Ley) $4.95

____ **Colostrum: Nature's Gift to the Immune System** (Ley) $5.95

____ **DHA: The Magnificent Marine Oil** (Ley) $6.95

____ **DHEA: Unlocking the Secrets/Fountain of Youth-2nd ed.** (Ash & Ley) . . .$14.95

____ **Diabetes to Wholeness** (Ley) $9.95

____ **Discover the Beta Glucan Secret** (Ley) $3.95

____ **Fading: One family's journey ... Alzheimer's** (Kraft) $12.95

____ **Flax! Fabulous Flax!** (Ley) $4.95

____ **Flax Lignans: Fifty Years to Harvest** (Sönju & Ley) $4.95

____ **God Wants You Well** (Ley) $14.95

____ **Health Benefits of Probiotics** (Dash) $4.95

____ **How Did We Get So Fat? 2nd Edition** (Susser & Ley) $8.95

____ **How to Fight Osteoporosis and Win!** (Ley) $6.95

____ **Maca: Adaptogen and Hormone Balancer (Ley)** $4.95

____ **Marvelous Memory Boosters** (Ley) $3.95

____ **Medicinal Mushrooms:** Agaricus Blazei Murill (Ley) $4.95

____ **MSM: On Our Way Back to Health W/ Sulfur** (Ley) SPANISH $3.95

____ **MSM: On Our Way Back to Health W/ Sulfur** (Ley) $4.95

____ **Natural Healing Handbook** (Ley) $14.95

Nature's Road to Recovery: Nutritional Supplements for the Alcoholic
____ **& Chemical Dependent** (Ley) $5.95

____ **PhytoNutrients: Medicinal Nutrients in Foods,** *Revised /Updated* (Ley) $5.95

____ **Recipes For Life! (Spiral Bound Cookbook)** (Ley) $19.95

____ **Secrets the Oil Companies Don't Want You to Know** (LaPointe) $10.00

Spewed! How to Cast Out Lukewarm Christianity through Fasting and a
____ **Fasted Lifestyle -** $15.95

____ **The Potato Antioxidant: Alpha Lipoic Acid** (Ley) $6.95

____ **Vinpocetine: Revitalize Your Brain w/ Periwinkle Extract!** (Ley) $4.95

Subtotal $ _____   Please add $5.00 for shipping. **TOTAL $** _____

Credit card orders call toll free: 1-877-BOOKS11

Also visit: www.blpublications.com